SKINUENTUREZ

WART-O-WEEN

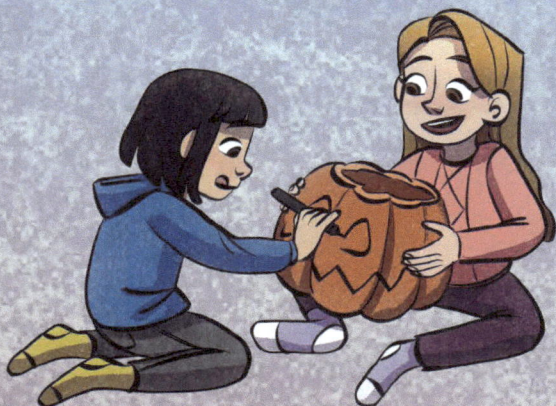

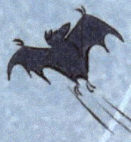

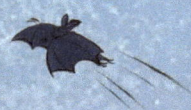

For permissions, please contact:
Skinventurez LLC
pr@skinventurez.com

SKINVENTUREZ: Wart-o-ween
Written by Dr. Tamara Lazic Strugar
Illustrated by Lea Embeli
Book design, lettering and production by Biljana Mihajlovic
Logo design by Melina Mikulic
Edited by Mia Strugar & Amy Betz
For inquiries or information regarding
this book, please contact:
www.skinventurez.com
pr@skinventurez.com

ISBN: 979-8-9887922-6-0

Disclaimer: The information contained in this book is
for educational purposes only and is not intended as a
substitute for professional medical advice, diagnosis,
or treatment. Always seek the advice of a qualified
healthcare provider with any questions you may
have regarding a medical condition. The author and
publisher are not liable for any actions taken or not
taken based on the information provided in this book.

Note: The information provided above is fictional and should
not be used as actual contact details for a publisher.

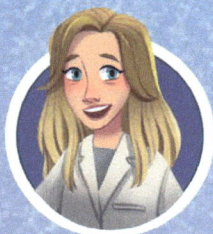

A GRAPHIC NOVEL BY
DR. TAMARA LAZIC STRUGAR

SKINVENTUREZ
Wart-o-ween

ILLUSTRATED BY
Lea Embeli

LETTERING AND DESIGN
Biljana Mihajlovic

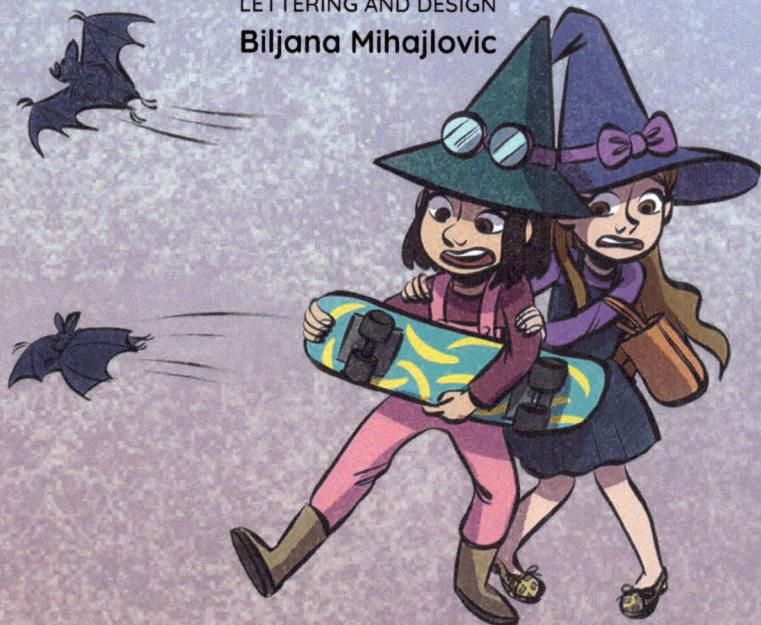

This book is dedicated to everyone who has supported me in my unexpected life journey- from doctor to patient, from dermatologist to book author...

A special thanks to my mini-me, Mia, my inspiration and main partner in this book project. And to Luka & John- my boys, the loves of my life.

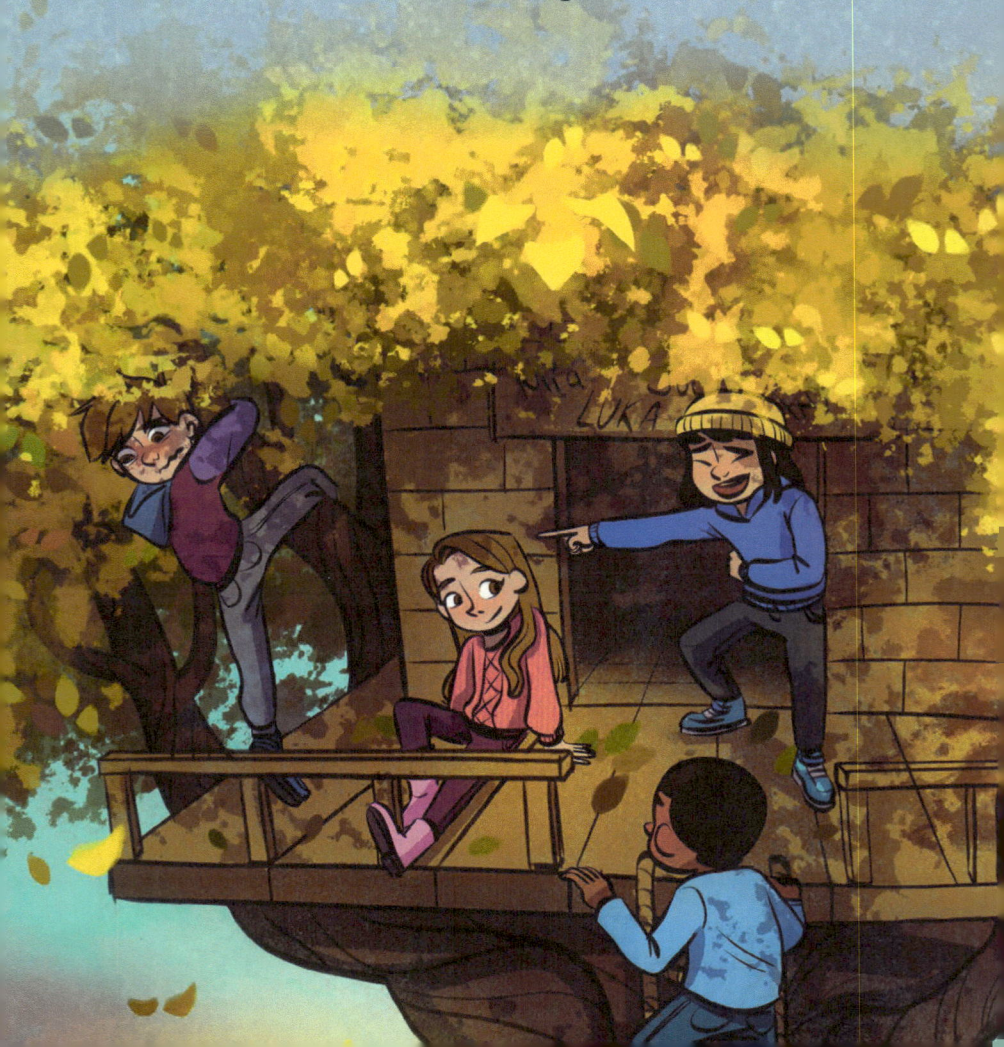

CHAPTER ONE

Secret Scratchies

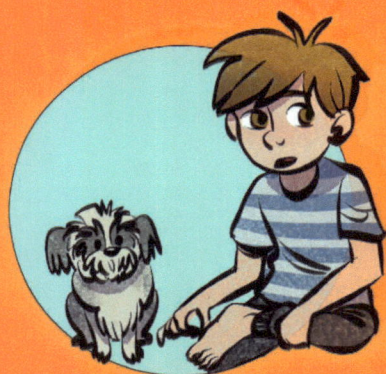

It was only a week till Halloween and Anya still didn't know if she could make it. It wouldn't be the same without her!

ANYA! Are you coming for **Halloween?**

Sorry, I can't. Mom and Dad are too busy.

Come with us then?! I'm sure it would be okay. Jude is coming too!

That would be **AWESOME!** I'll ask. GTG, the skatepark awaits!

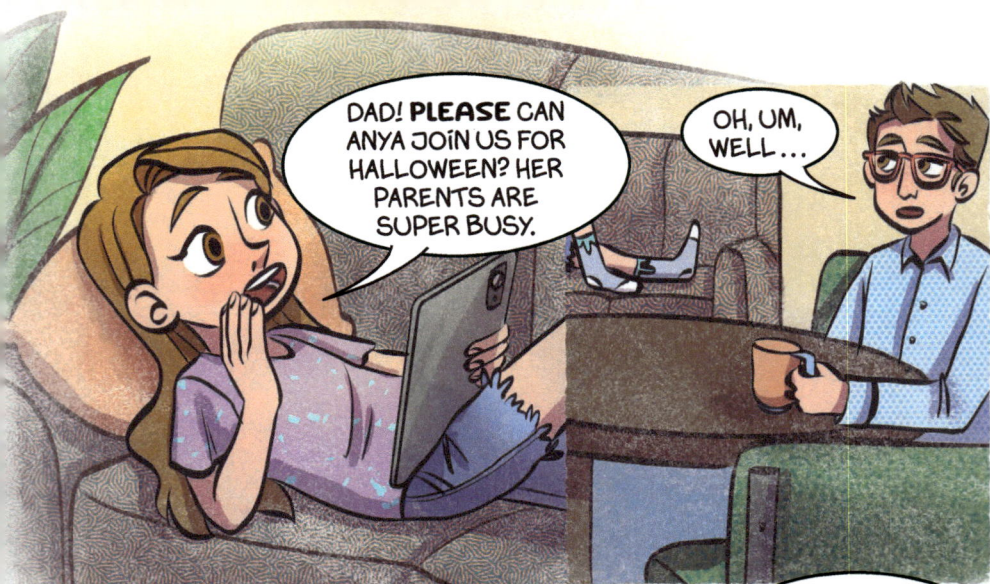

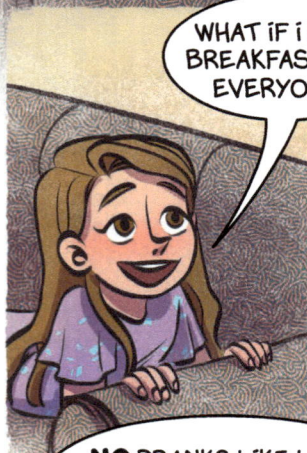

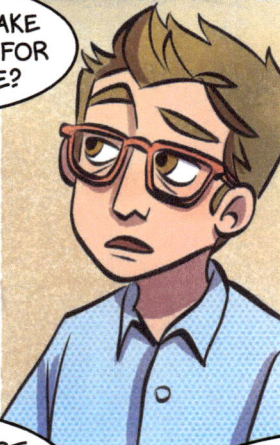

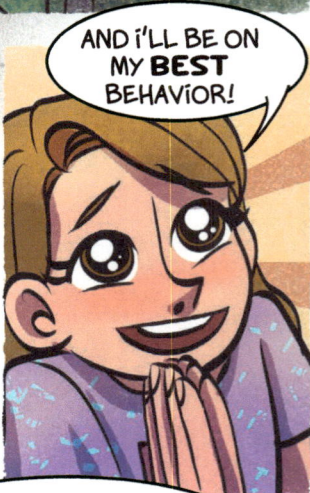

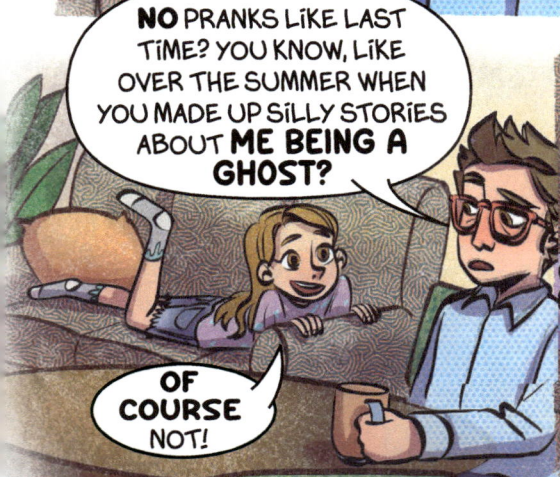

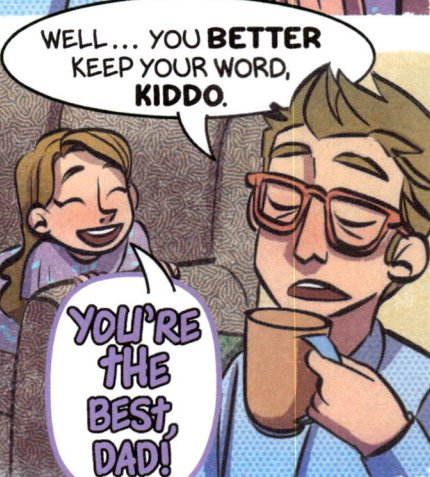

I had completely forgotten about Dad swallowing a ghost when we drove past the cemetery this summer. And pranking the boys into thinking he was a ghost. What a sunscreaming summer that was!

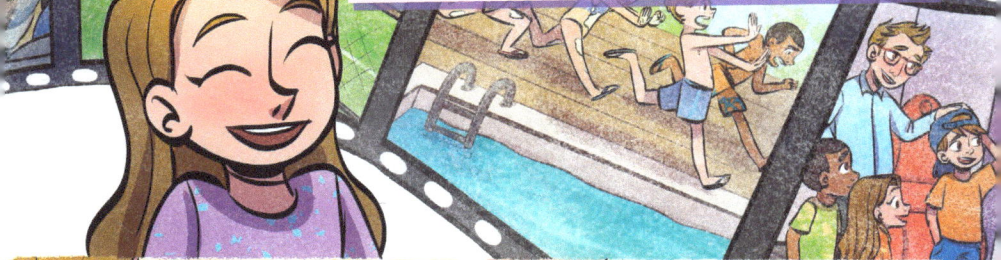

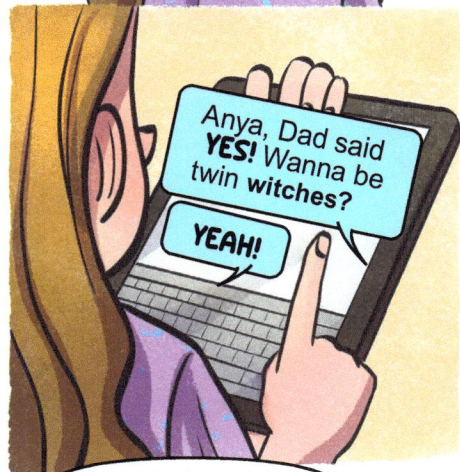

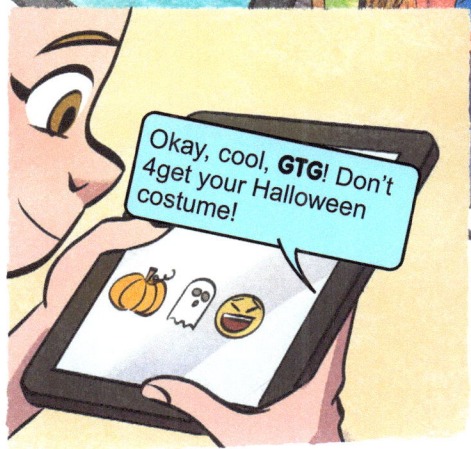

Anya, Dad said **YES!** Wanna be twin **witches**?

YEAH!

Okay, cool, **GTG**! Don't 4get your Halloween costume!

NOW WHERE IS THAT **WITCH'S HAT** i WORE WHEN i WAS iN MY HARRY POTTER PHASE?

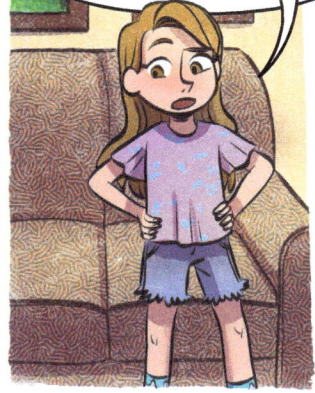

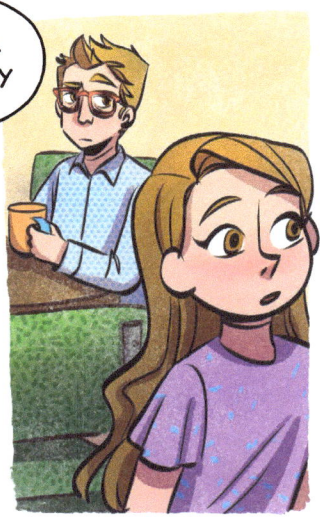

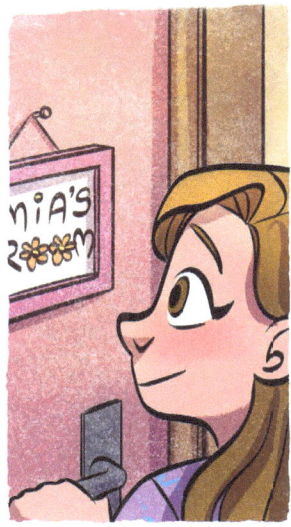

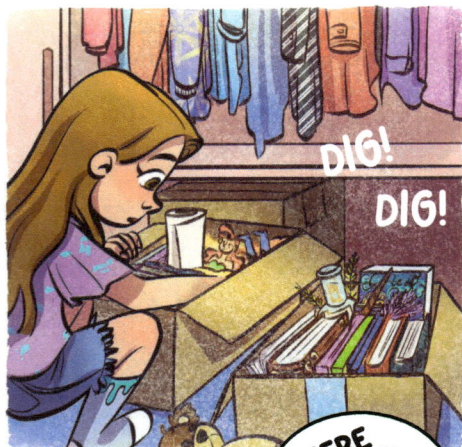

DIG!

DIG!

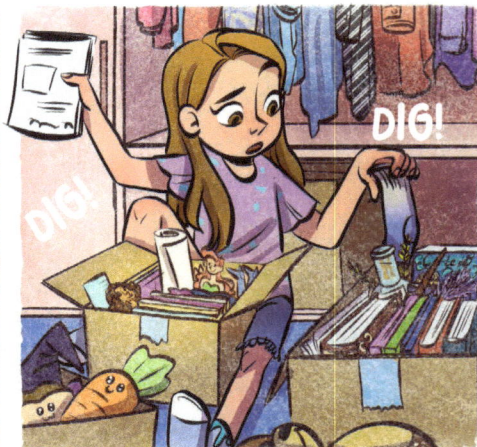

DIG!

DIG!

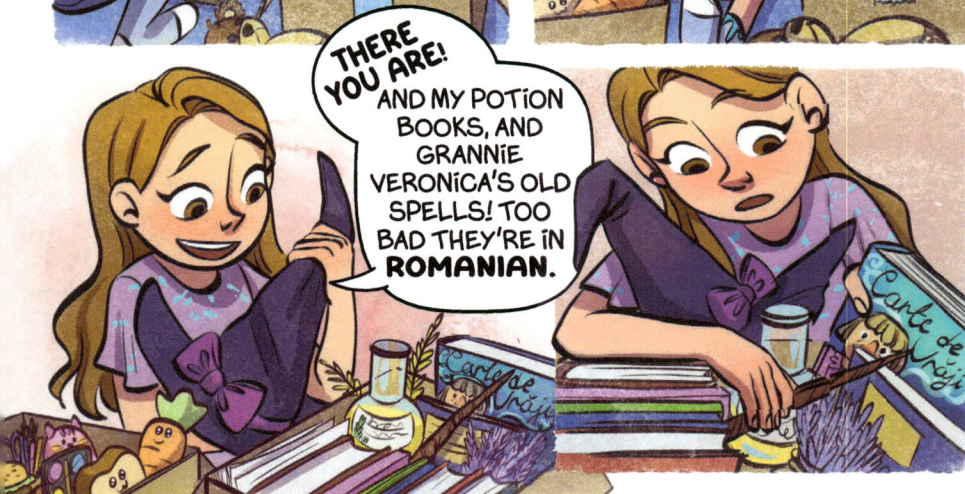

THERE YOU ARE! AND MY POTION BOOKS, AND GRANNIE VERONICA'S OLD SPELLS! TOO BAD THEY'RE IN **ROMANIAN.**

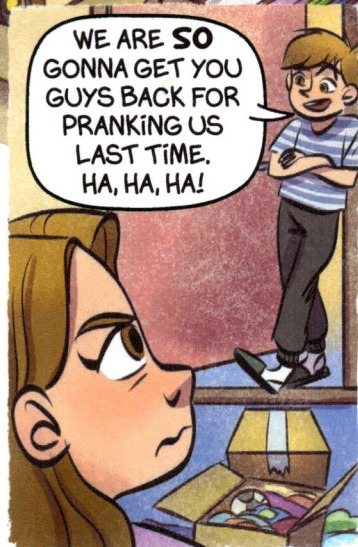

WE ARE **SO** GONNA GET YOU GUYS BACK FOR PRANKING US LAST TIME. HA, HA, HA!

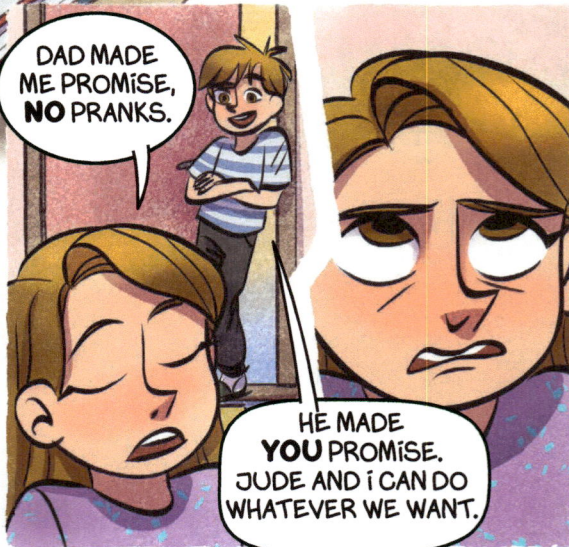

DAD MADE ME PROMISE, **NO** PRANKS.

HE MADE **YOU** PROMISE. JUDE AND I CAN DO WHATEVER WE WANT.

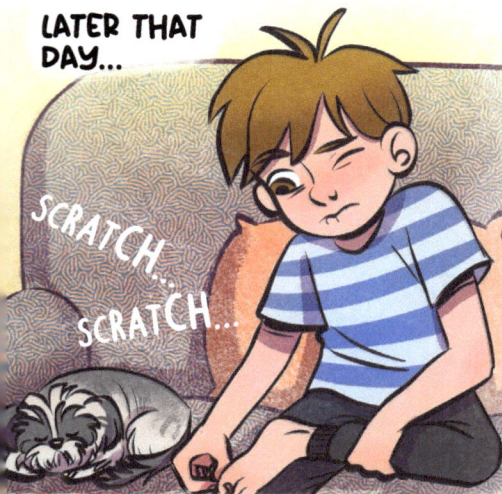

LATER THAT DAY...

SCRATCH...

SCRATCH...

WHAT'S **WRONG** WITH YOUR FEET? WHAT'S WITH THE SCRATCHING?

ER, NOTHING.

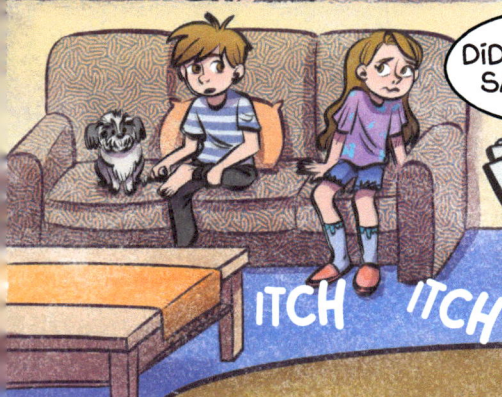

DID SOMEONE SAY **ITCH?**

ITCH ITCH

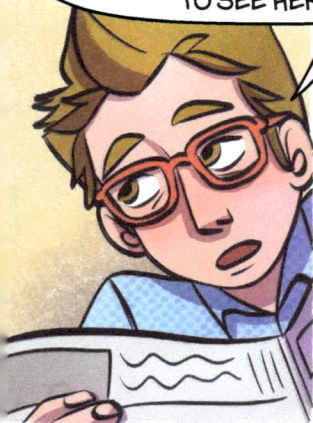

IF IT'S A SKIN CONDITION, I SHOULD CALL DR. LAZIC'S OFFICE RIGHT AWAY. I MIGHT BE ABLE TO GET A CHANCE TO SEE HER, I MEAN FOR **YOU** TO SEE HER...

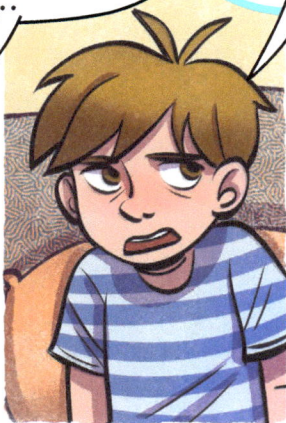

DAD!

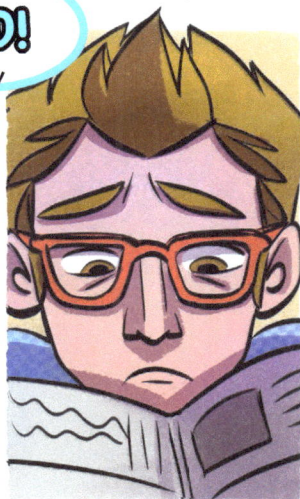

It was so good to be back in our country home!

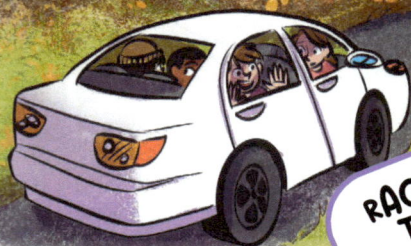

RACE YOU TO THE TREEHOUSE!

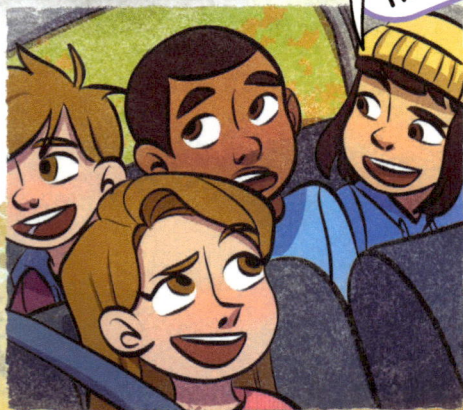

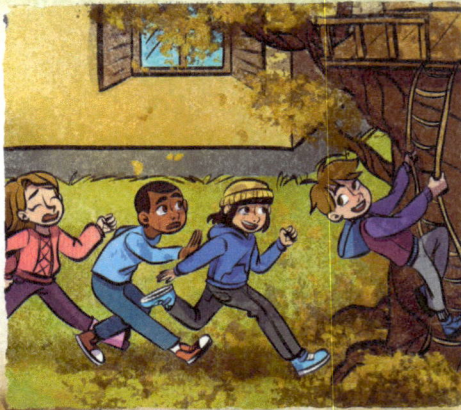

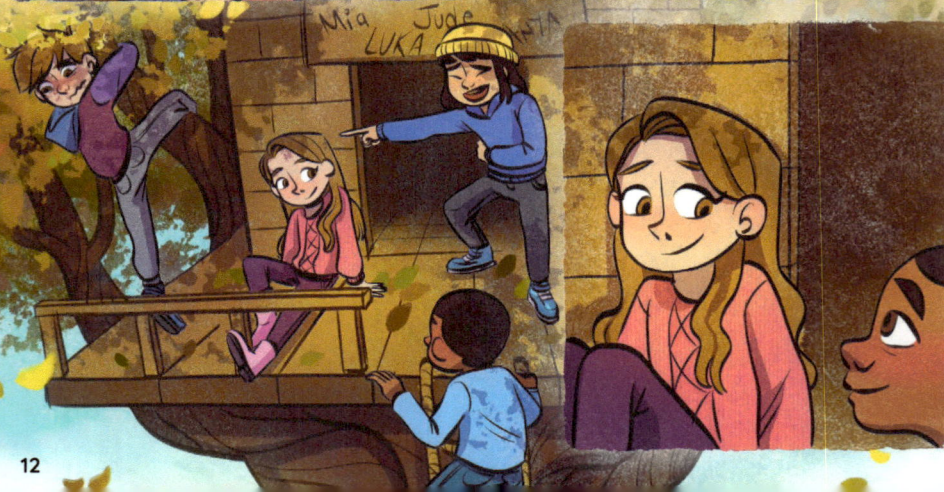

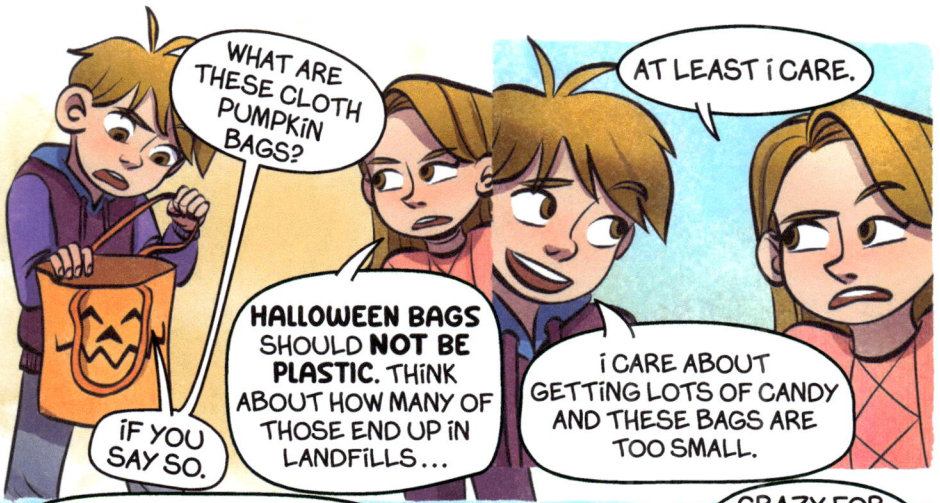

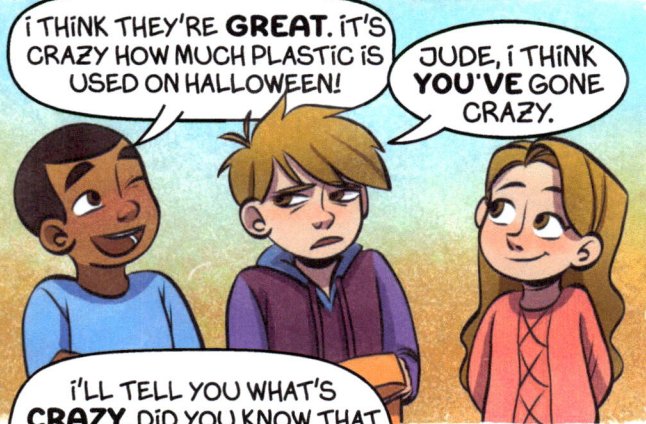

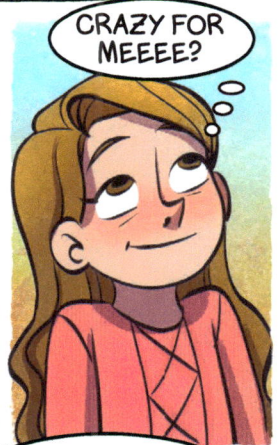

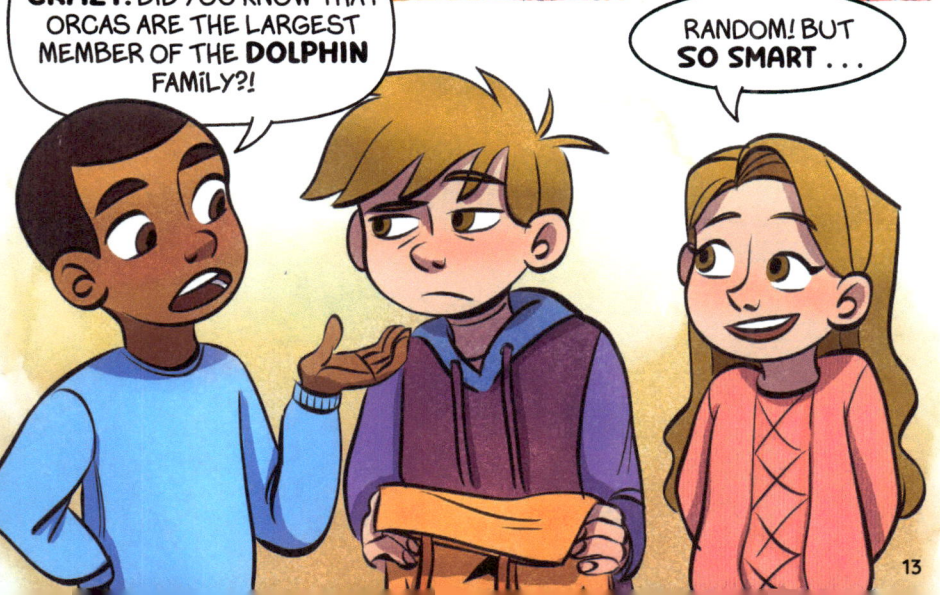

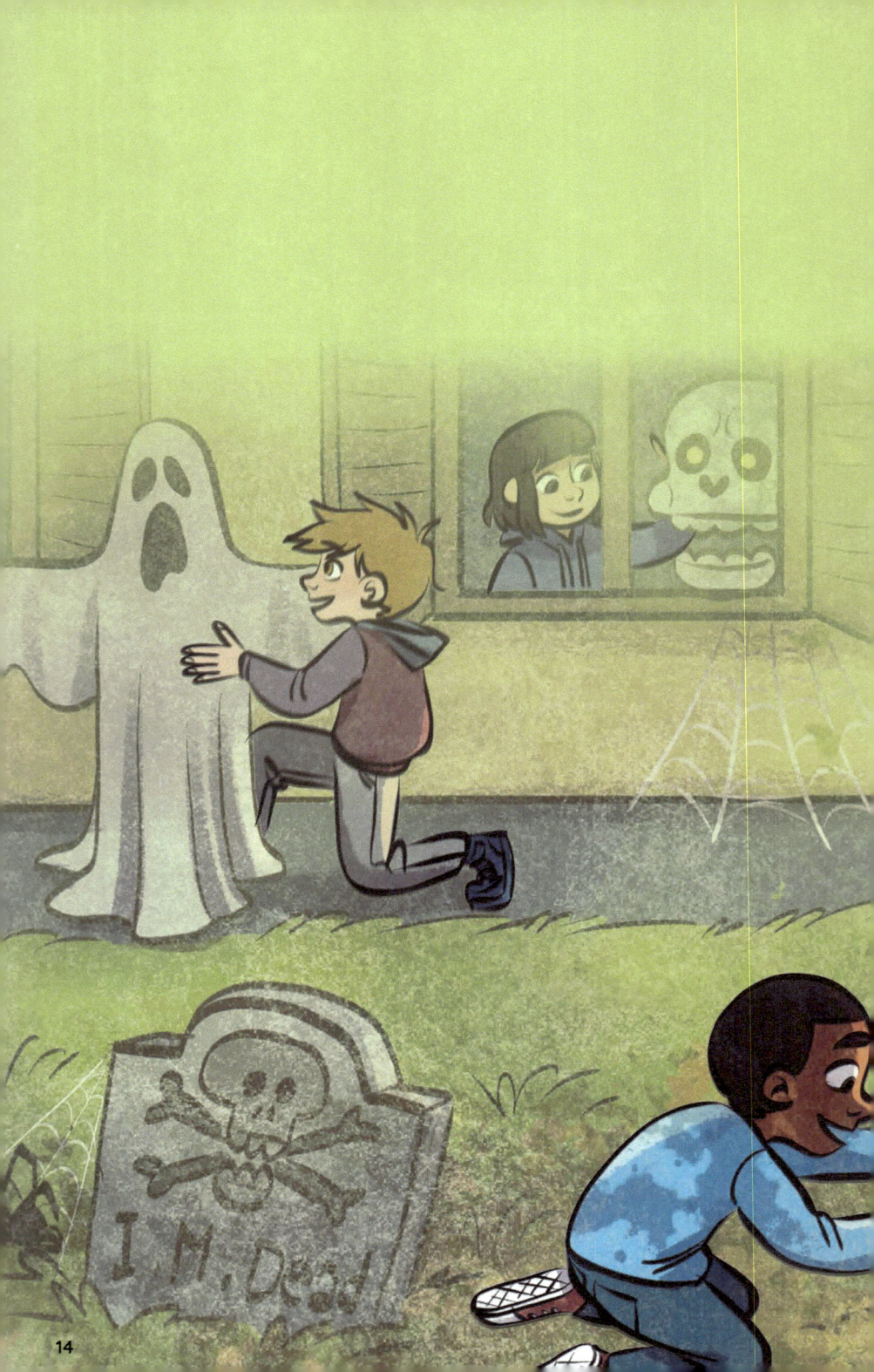

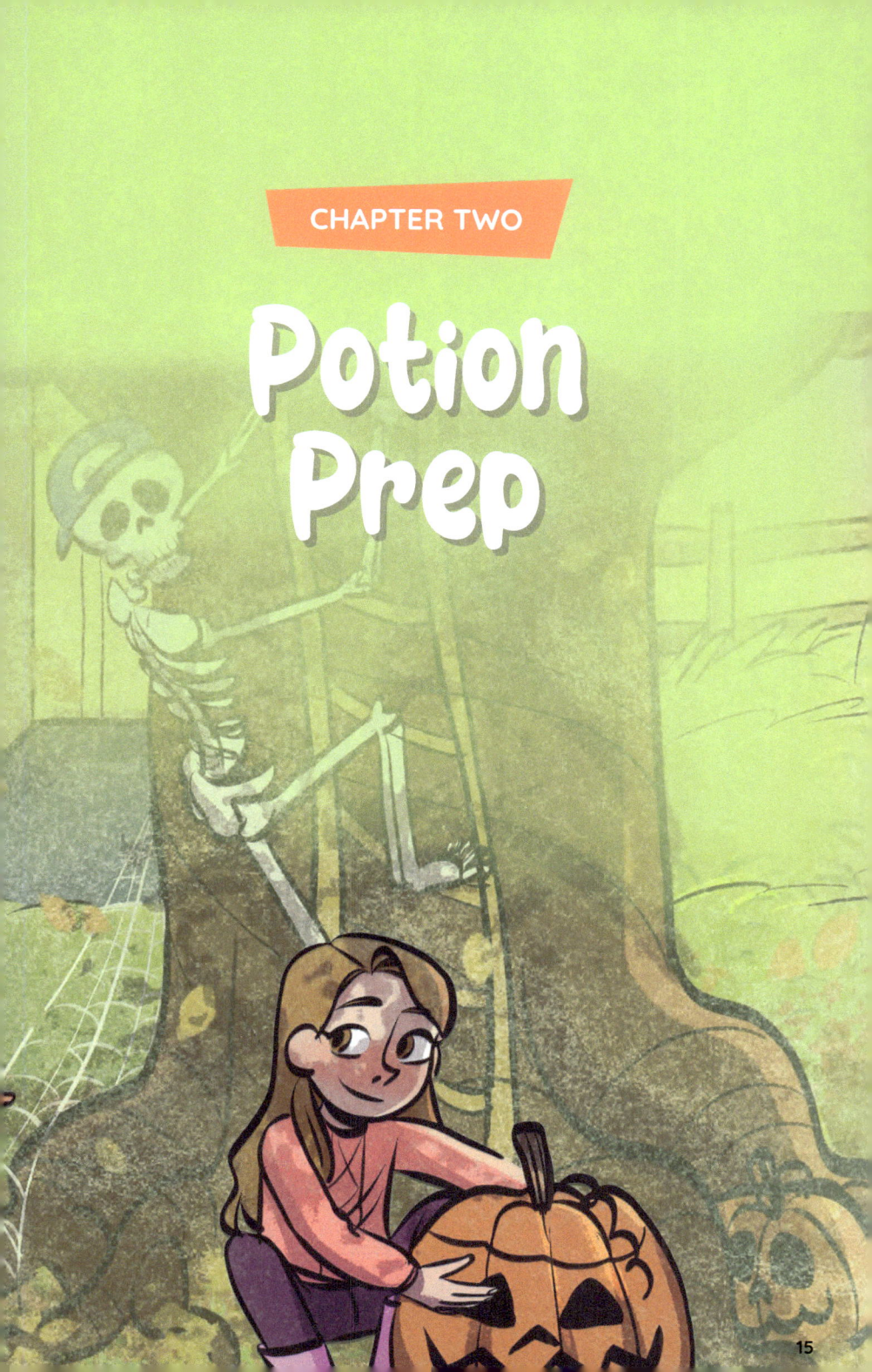

CHAPTER TWO

Potion Prep

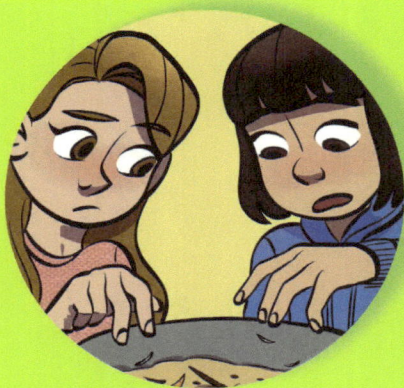

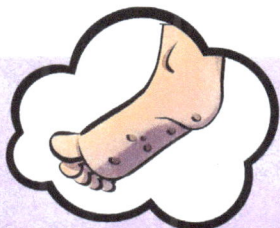

17

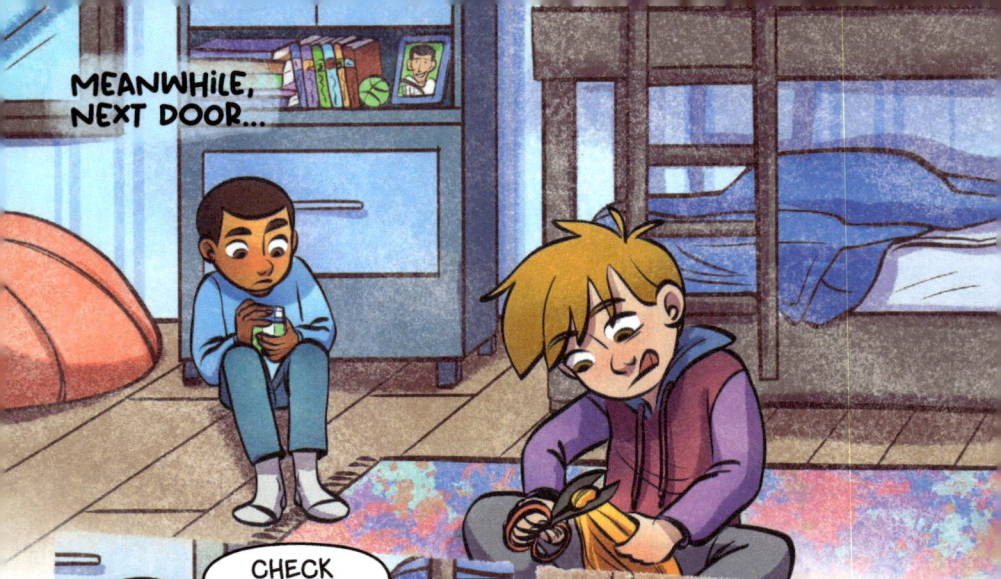

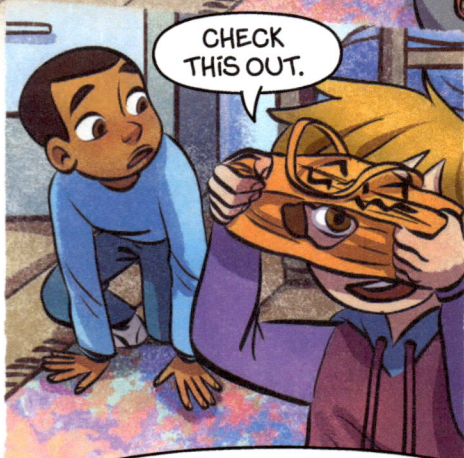

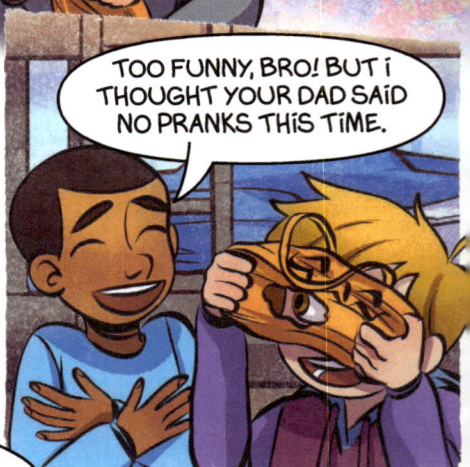

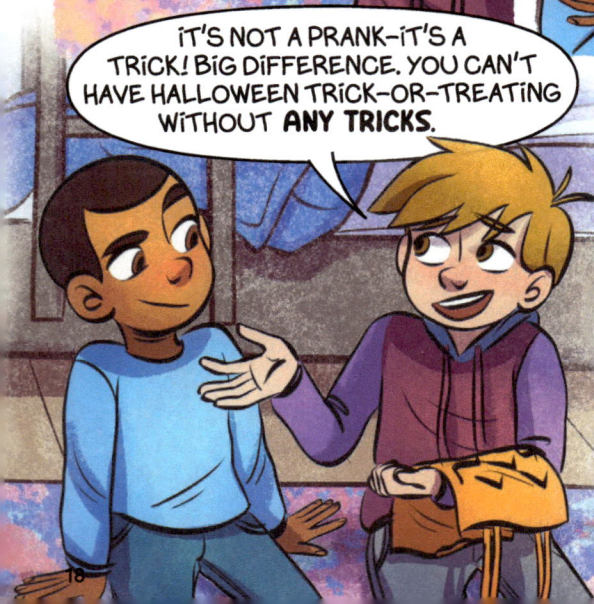

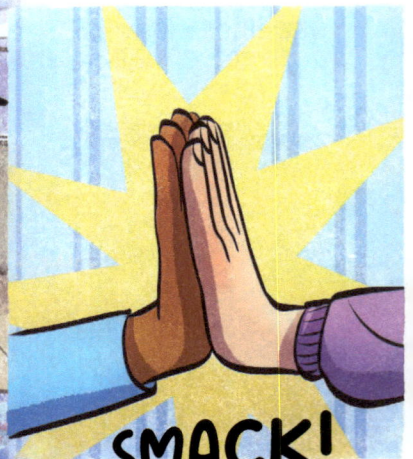

ITCHY, RED BUMPS... **LOOK, ANYA!** I'M PRETTY SURE **HE'S GOT WARTS!**

THERE ARE A FEW THINGS, BUT NOTHING WE COULD DO WITHOUT HIM KNOWING, UNLESS...

SO HOW DO WE GET RID OF THEM?

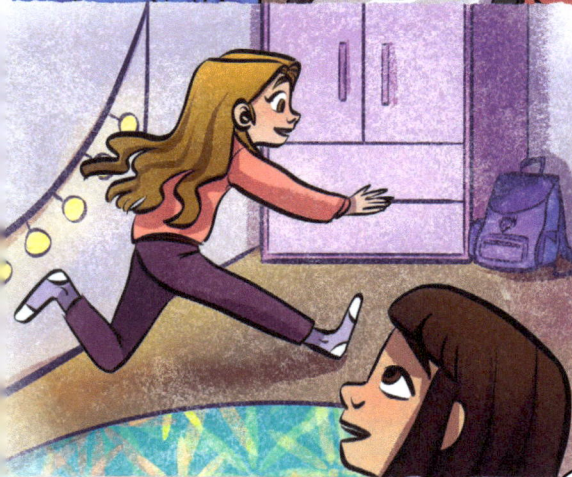

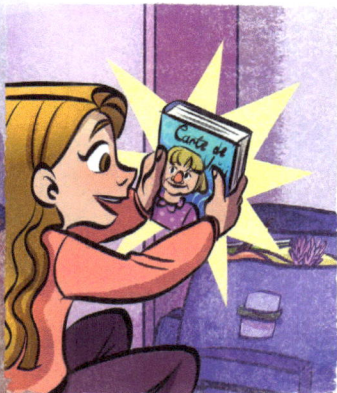

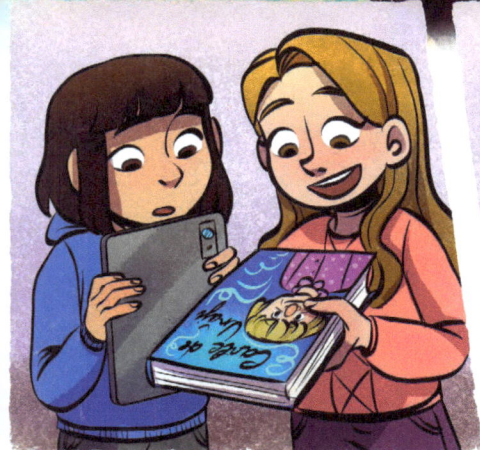

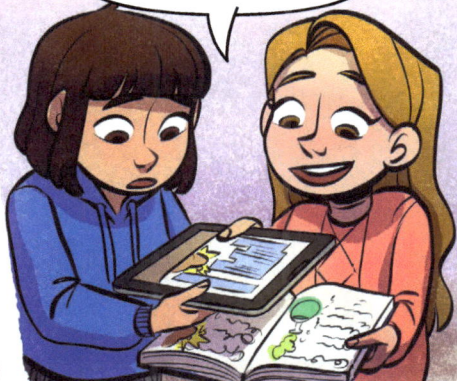

ROMANIAN TRANSLATOR APP TO THE RESCUE!

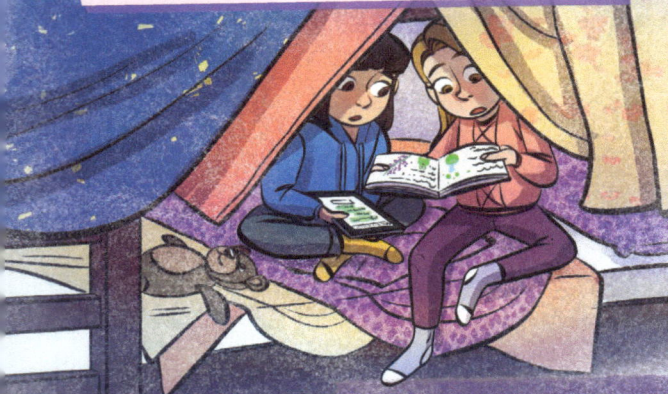

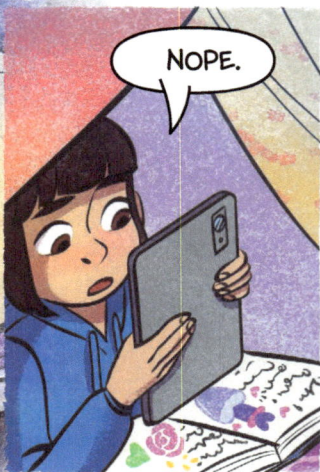

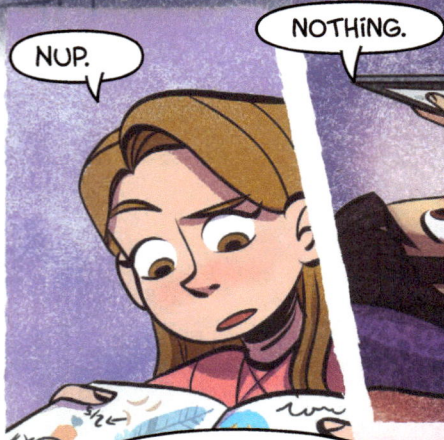

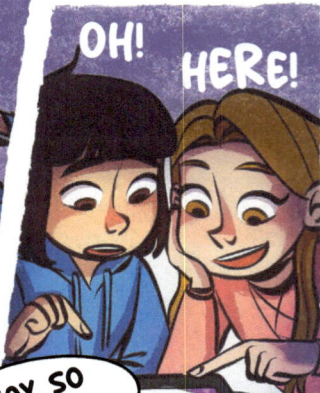

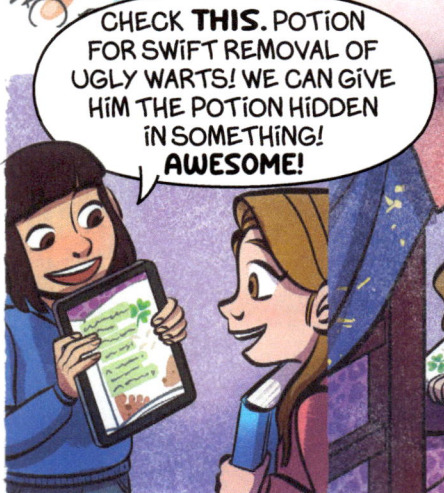

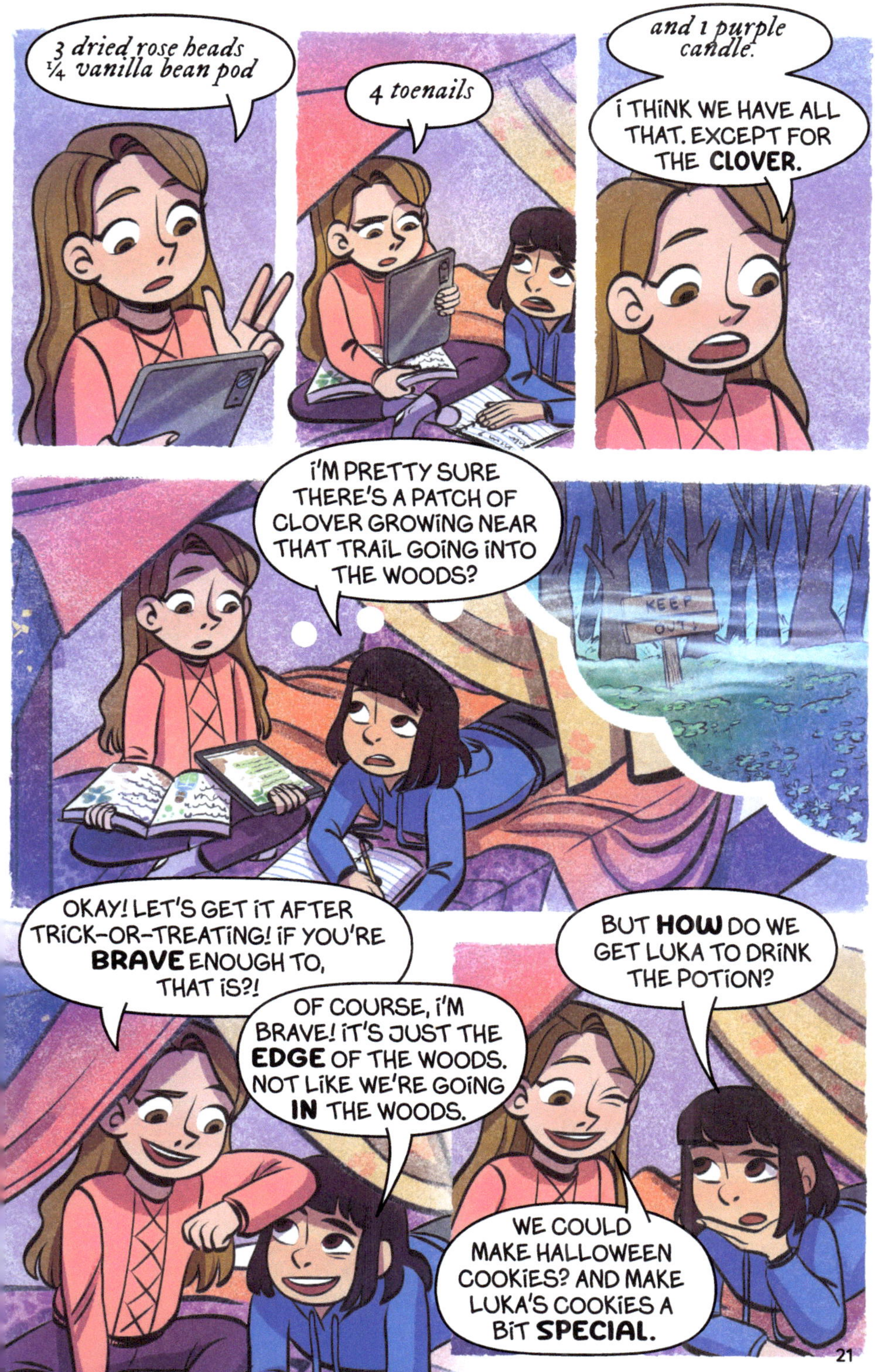
3 dried rose heads 1/4 vanilla bean pod
4 toenails
and 1 purple candle.
I THINK WE HAVE ALL THAT. EXCEPT FOR THE CLOVER.
I'M PRETTY SURE THERE'S A PATCH OF CLOVER GROWING NEAR THAT TRAIL GOING INTO THE WOODS?
KEEP OUT
OKAY! LET'S GET IT AFTER TRICK-OR-TREATING! IF YOU'RE BRAVE ENOUGH TO, THAT IS?!
OF COURSE, I'M BRAVE! IT'S JUST THE EDGE OF THE WOODS. NOT LIKE WE'RE GOING IN THE WOODS.
BUT HOW DO WE GET LUKA TO DRINK THE POTION?
WE COULD MAKE HALLOWEEN COOKIES? AND MAKE LUKA'S COOKIES A BIT SPECIAL.

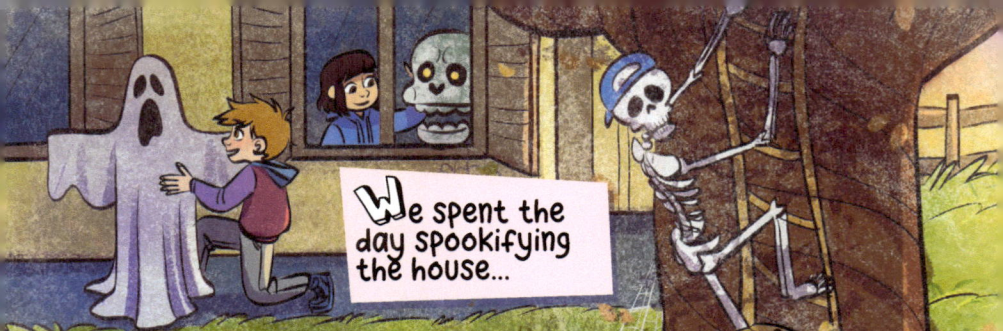

We spent the day spookifying the house...

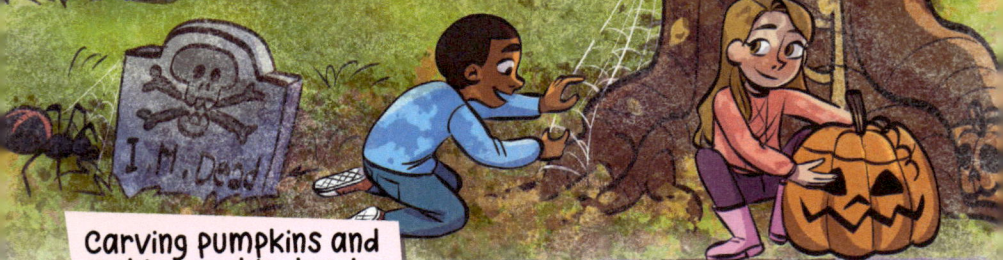

Carving pumpkins and making cookie dough.

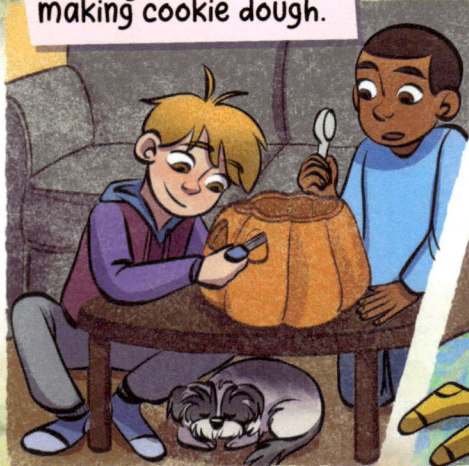

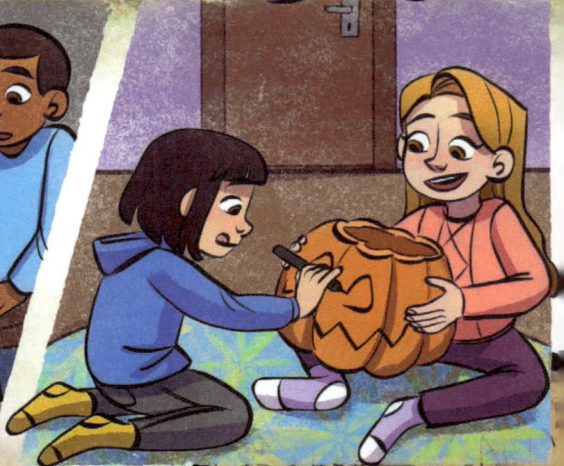

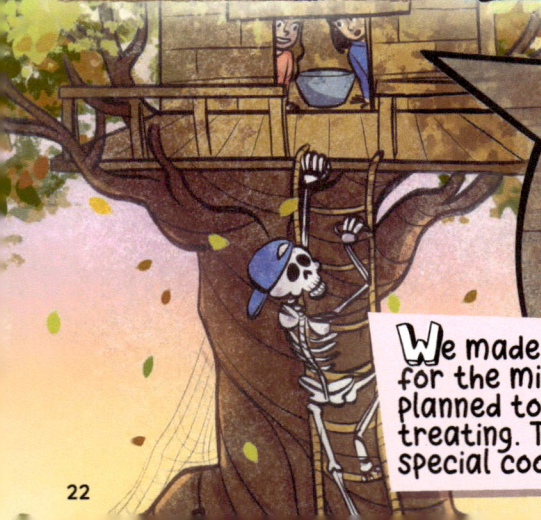

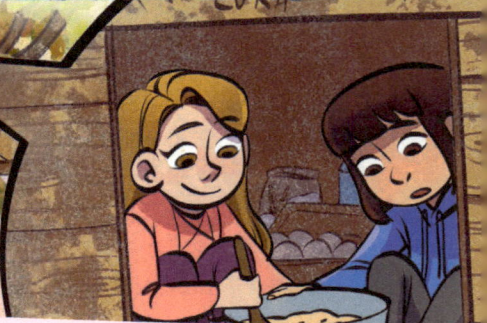

We made sure everything was ready for the missing ingredient that we planned to mix in after trick-or-treating. Then, we could give Luka the special cookies ASAP!

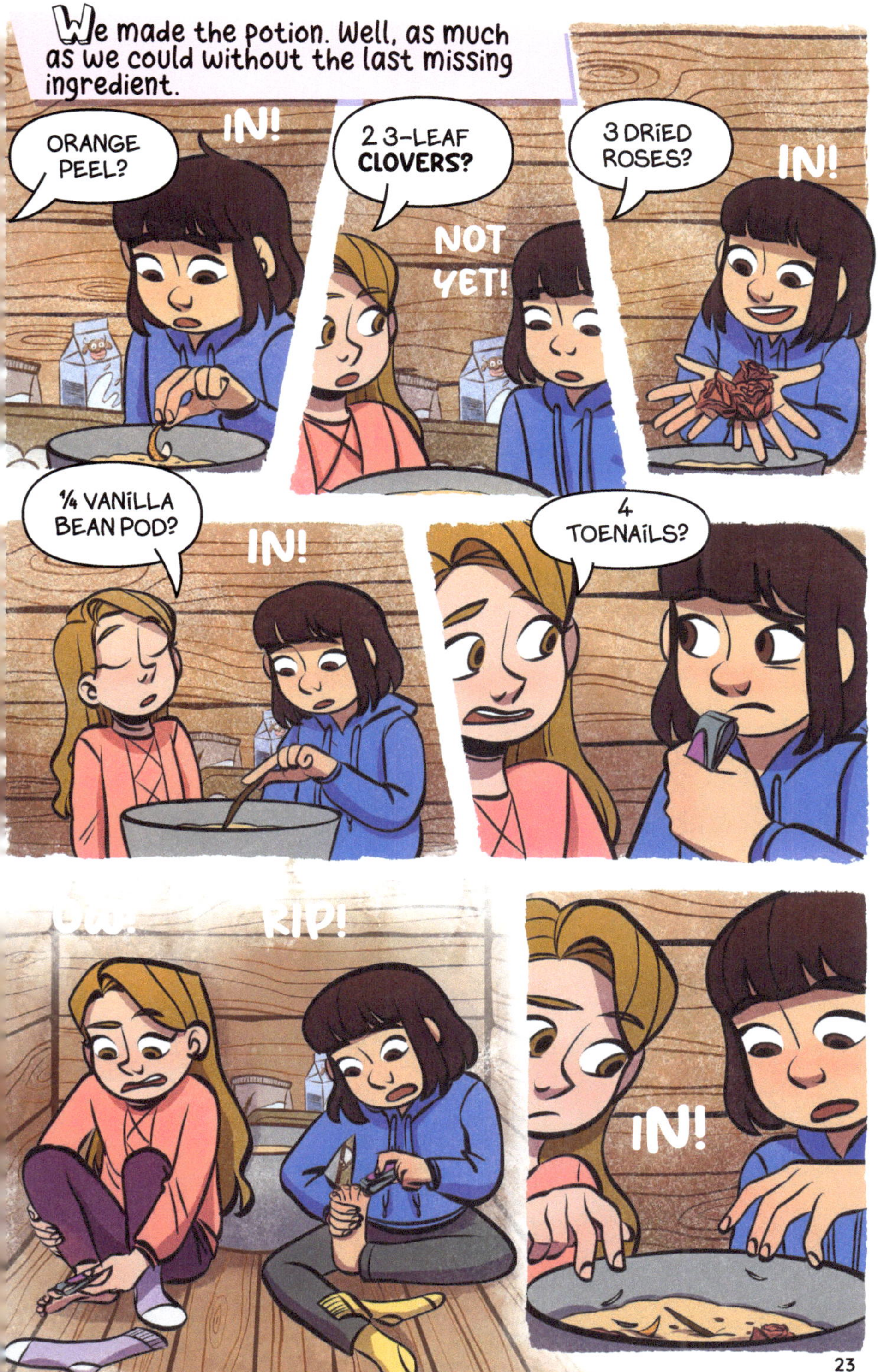
We made the potion. Well, as much as we could without the last missing ingredient.
ORANGE PEEL?
IN!
2 3-LEAF CLOVERS?
NOT YET!
3 DRIED ROSES?
IN!
¼ VANILLA BEAN POD?
IN!
4 TOENAILS?
OW!
RIP!
IN!

Then we figured out our costumes.

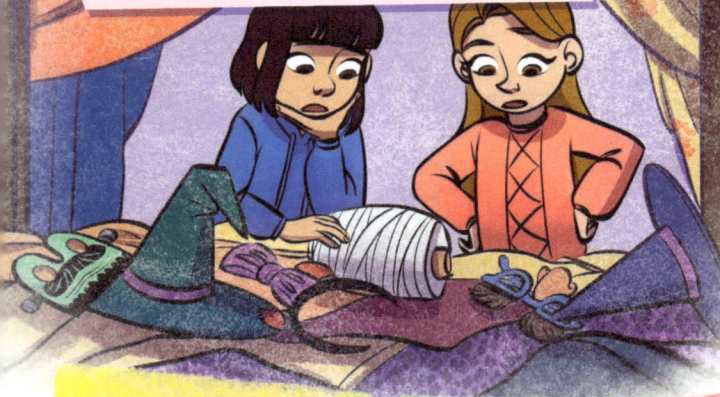

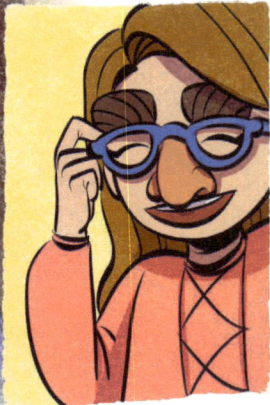

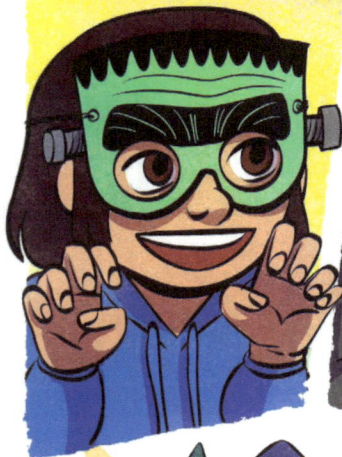

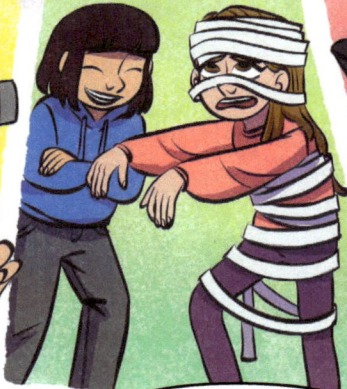

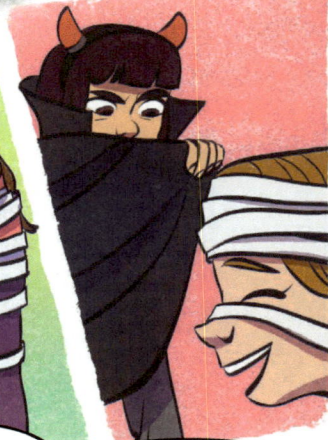

YOU CAN'T **NOT** WEAR THOSE HEELS FOR ONCE?

OF COURSE, I WON'T **NOT** WEAR THEM FOR ONCE!

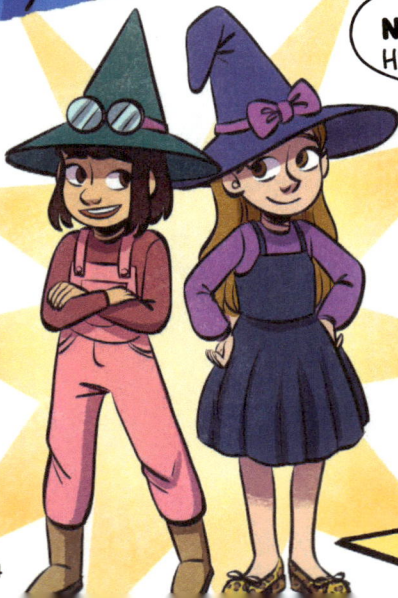

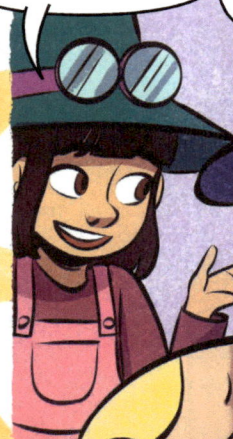

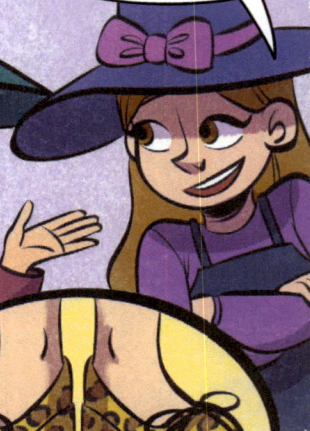

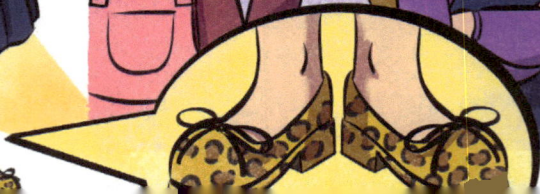

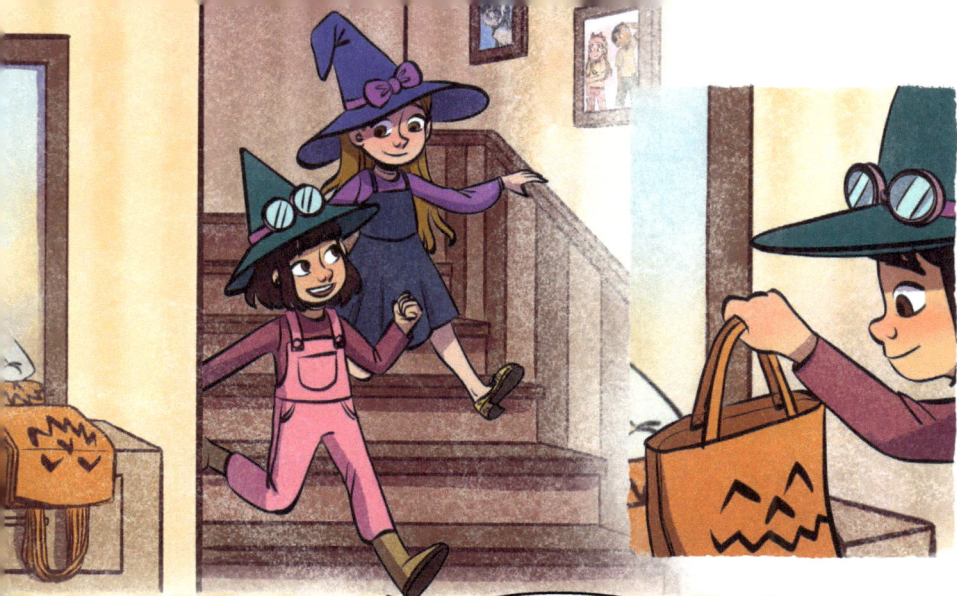

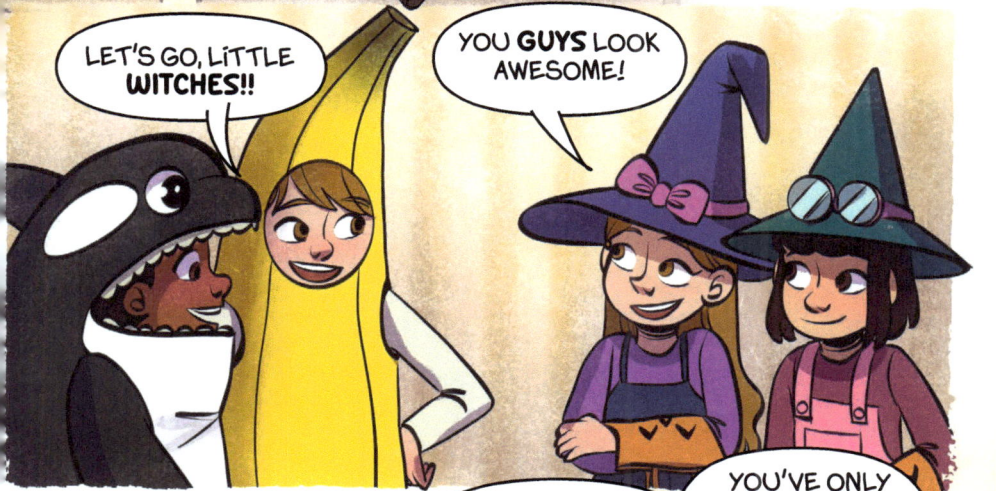

LET'S GO, LITTLE **WITCHES**!!

YOU **GUYS** LOOK AWESOME!

HEY, DID YOU KNOW THAT AN **ORCA** IS ALMOST AS BIG AS A **BUS?**

YOU'VE ONLY TOLD US THAT, LIKE **THREE** TIMES ALREADY.

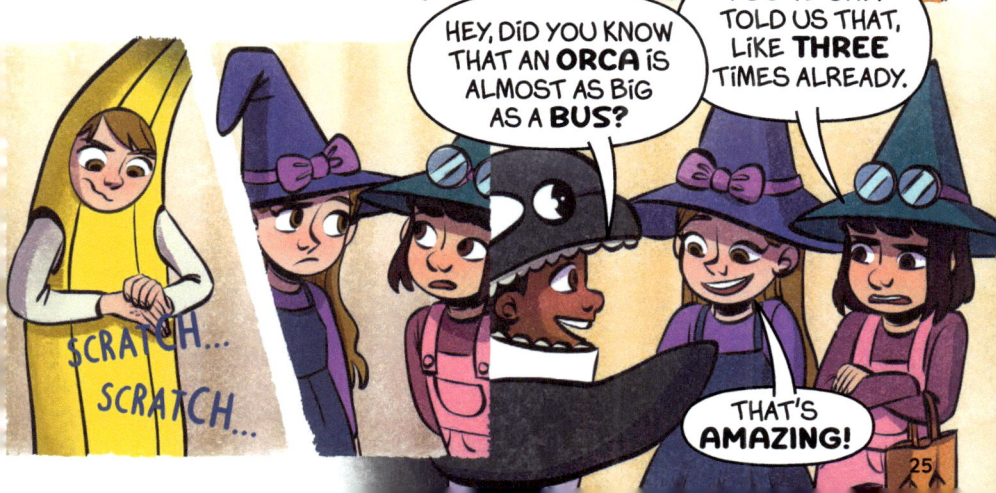

SCRATCH...

SCRATCH...

THAT'S **AMAZING!**

BYE, MR. DAD!

BYE, DAD!

HEY, GUYS, WAIT FOR ME!

OH, C'MON, DAD! WE'LL LOOK LIKE SILLY LITTLE **KIDS** IF WE HAVE YOU WITH US.

BUT YOU **ARE** MY SILLY LITTLE KIDDOS!

DADS LOVE CANDY TOO!

PLUS, YOU WON'T EVEN KNOW I'M THERE, UNLESS I CREEP UP BEHIND YOU AND ... **BOO!**

YOUR DAD **SO** MAKES A GOOD GHOST. STILL FREAKS ME OUT WHEN I REMEMBER WE THOUGHT HE WAS A REAL GHOST!

FINE.

I **KNOW!** ALL THAT DRAMA OVER DAD USING TOO MUCH SUNSCREEN!

Connecticut looks amazing this time of the year.

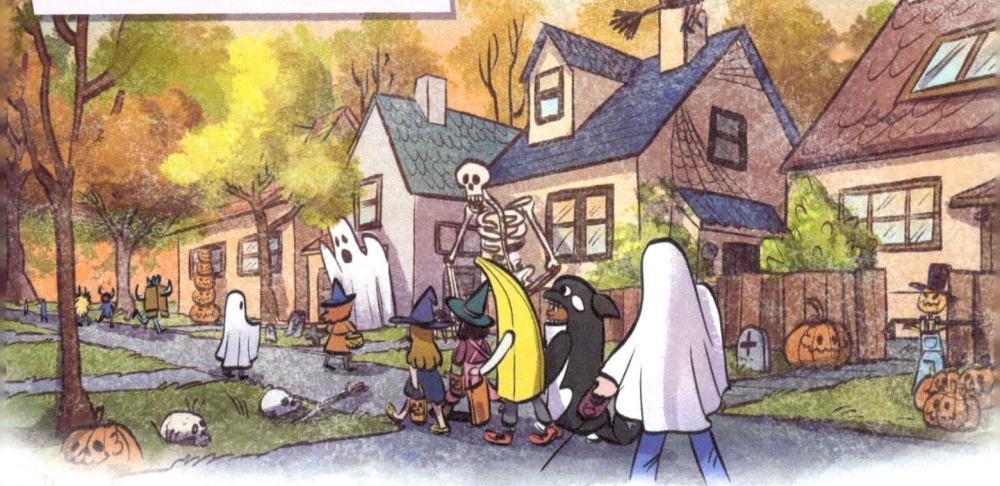

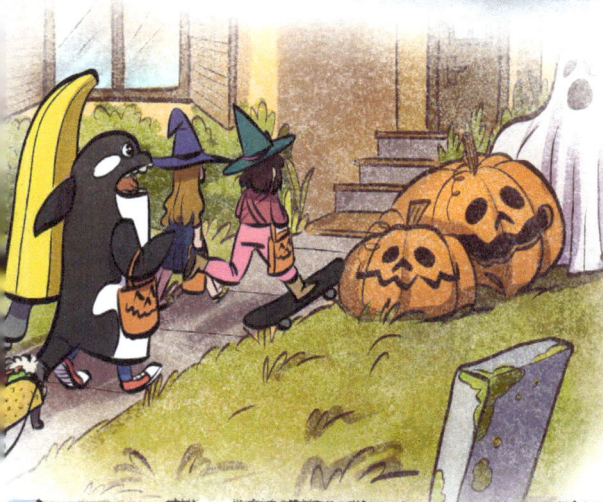

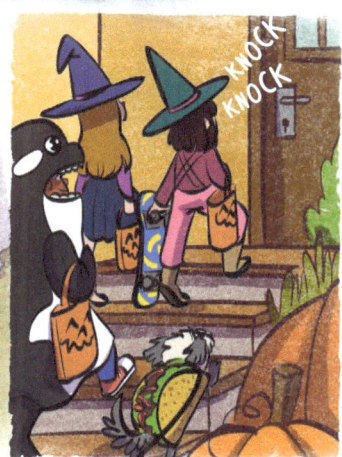

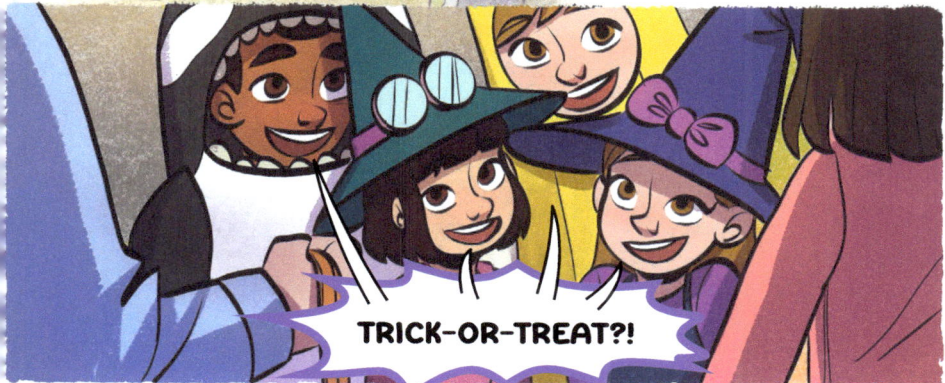

KNOCK KNOCK

TRICK-OR-TREAT?!

We saw LOADS of spooky stuff.

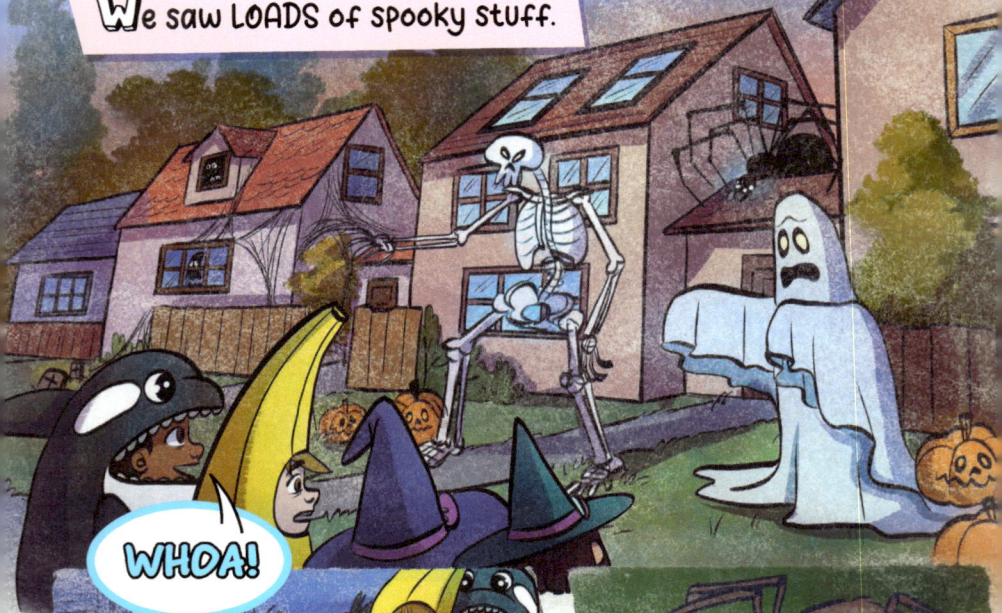

WHOA!

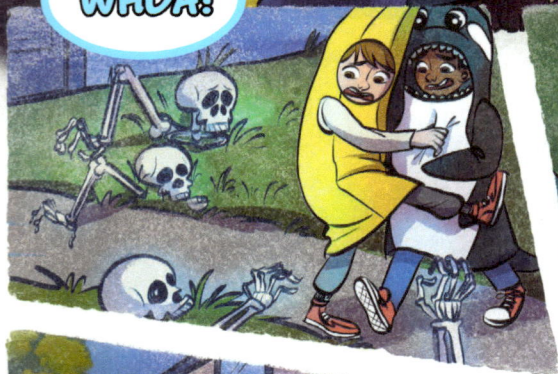

EW! THAT'S **TOO** MUCH!

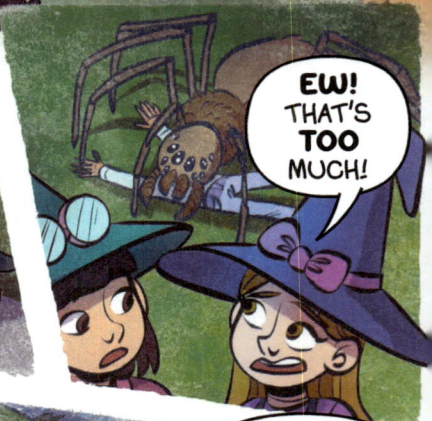

AWESOME!

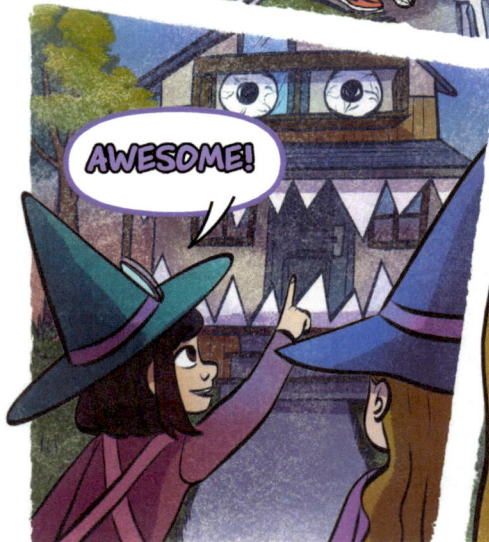

THAT PUMPKIN LOOKS **SERIOUSLY** MEAN!

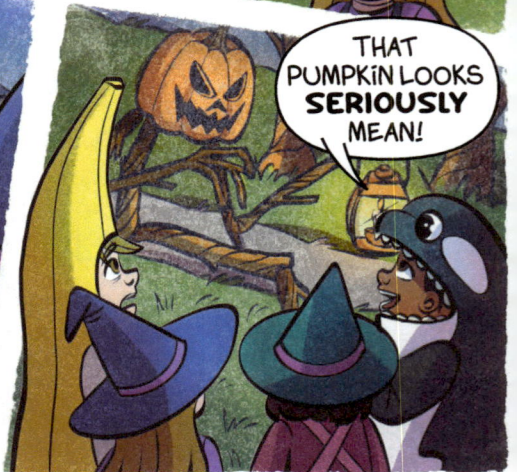

And we got LOADS of yummy stuff.

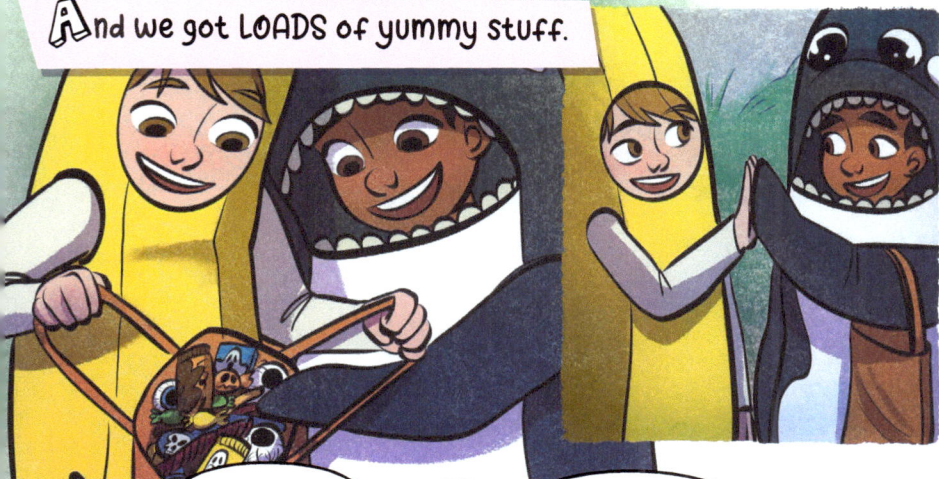

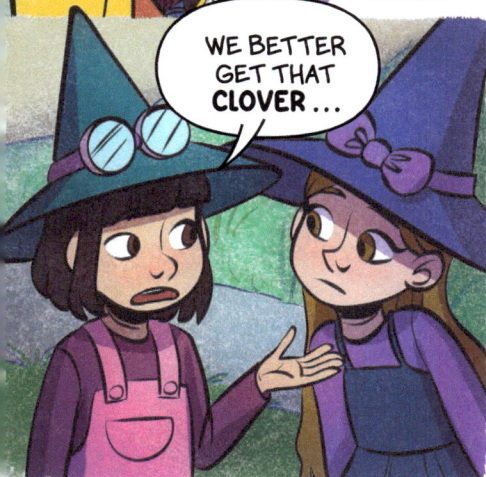

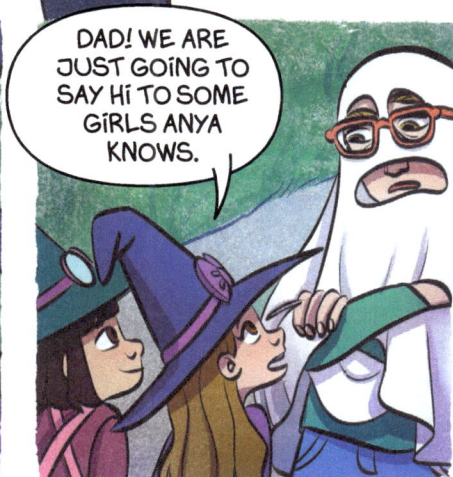

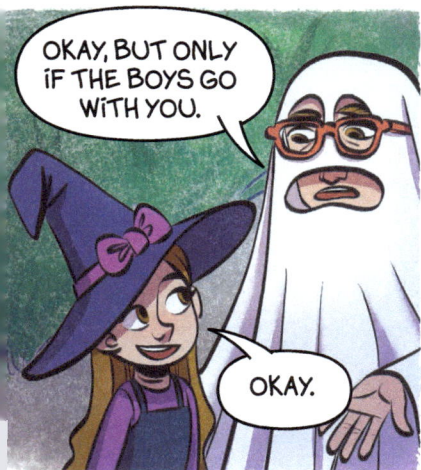

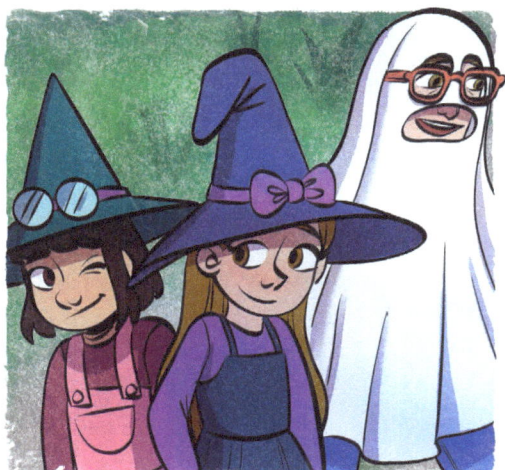

WE BETTER GET THAT **CLOVER** ...

DAD! WE ARE JUST GOING TO SAY HI TO SOME GIRLS ANYA KNOWS.

OKAY, BUT ONLY IF THE BOYS GO WITH YOU.

OKAY.

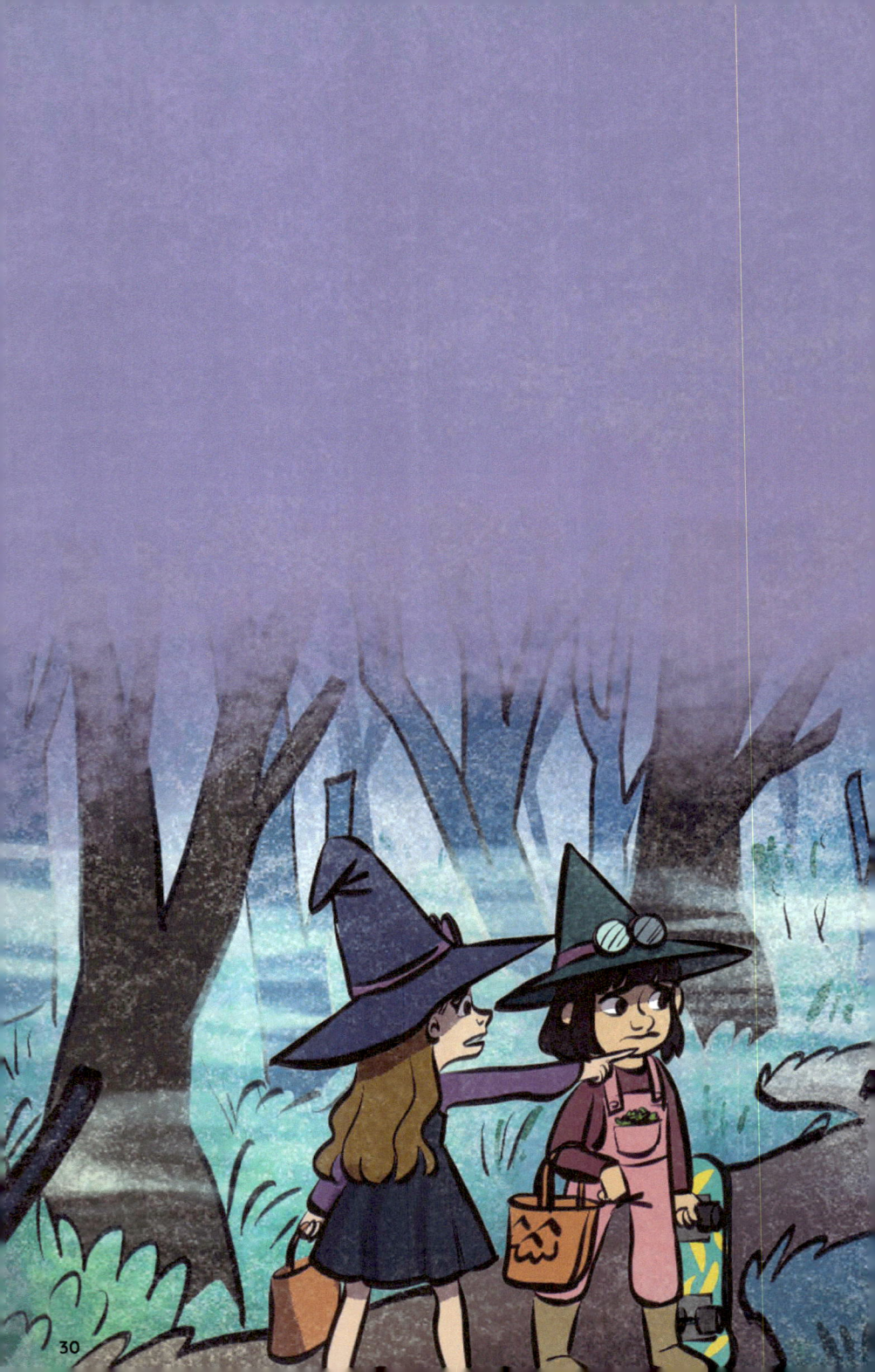

CHAPTER THREE

Peek and Freak

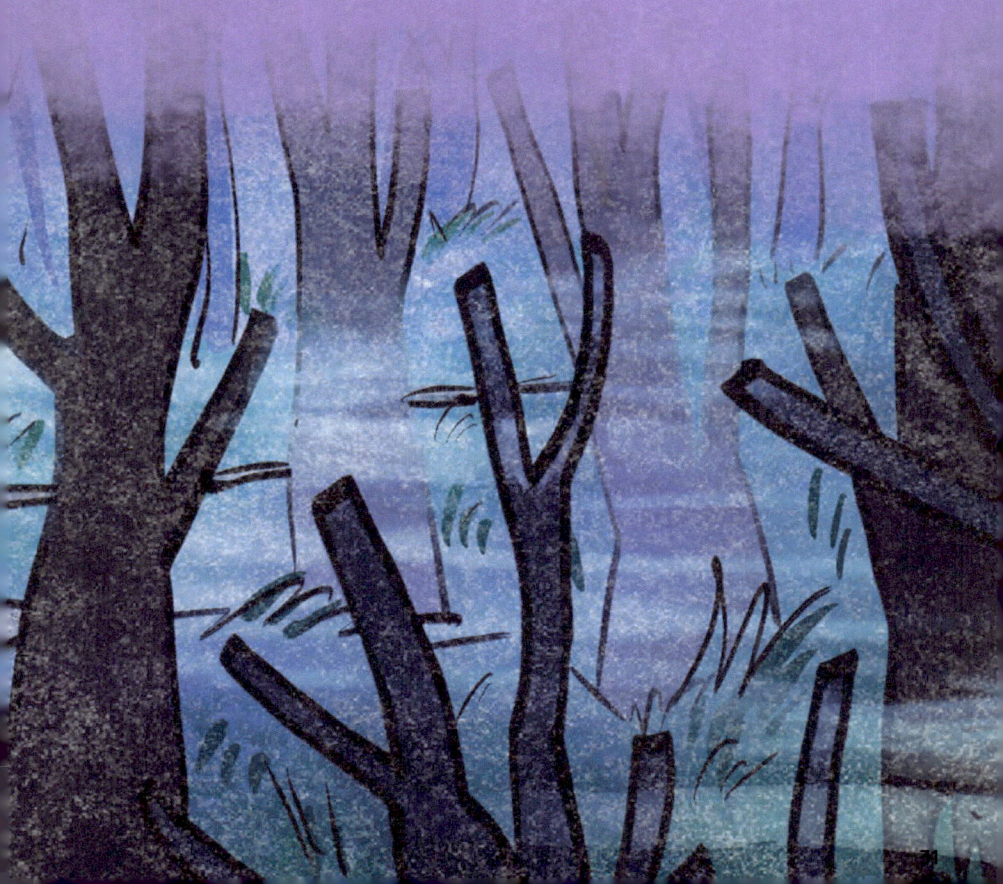

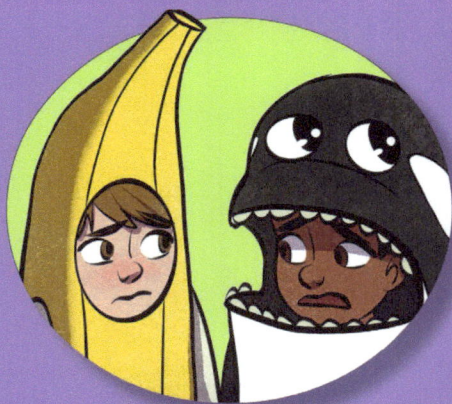

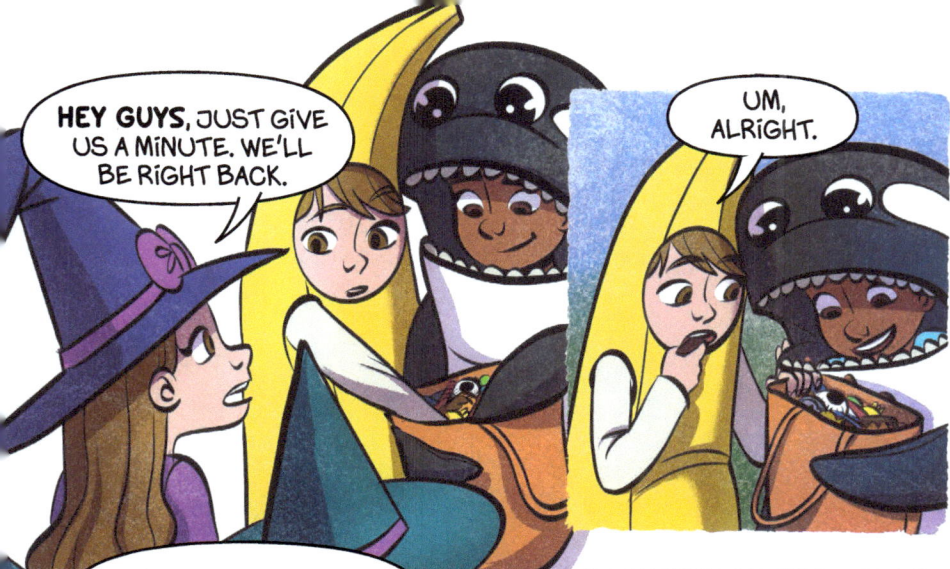

HEY GUYS, JUST GIVE US A MINUTE. WE'LL BE RIGHT BACK.

UM, ALRIGHT.

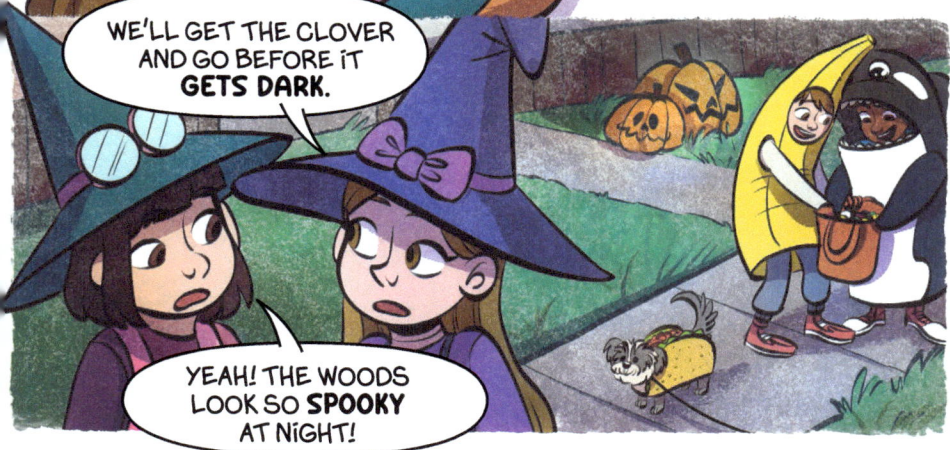

WE'LL GET THE CLOVER AND GO BEFORE IT **GETS DARK**.

YEAH! THE WOODS LOOK SO **SPOOKY** AT NIGHT!

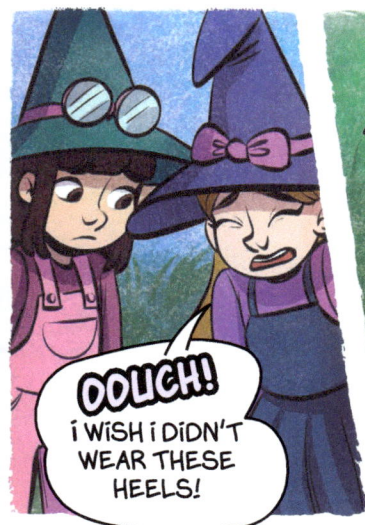

OOUCH! I WISH I DIDN'T WEAR THESE HEELS!

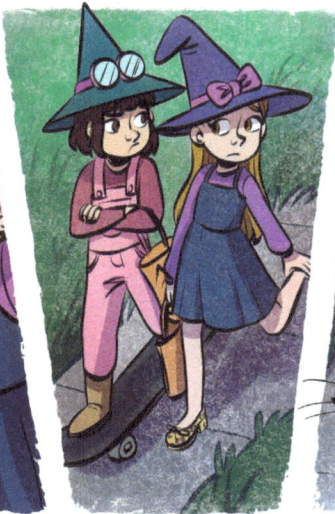

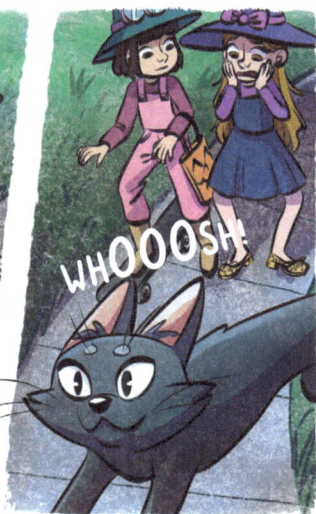

WHOOOSH!

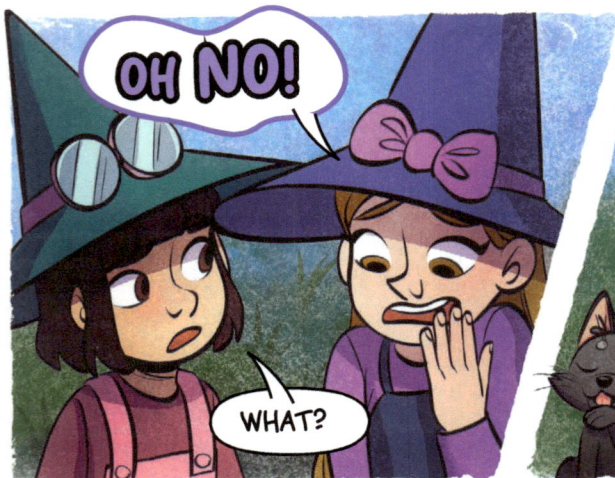

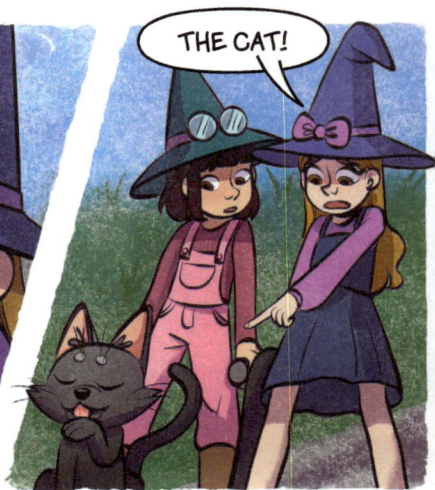

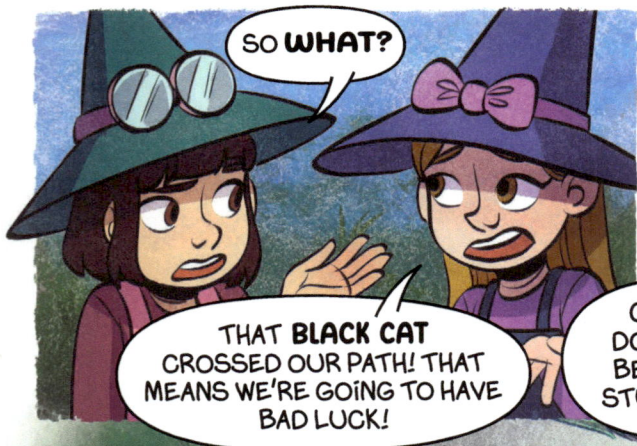

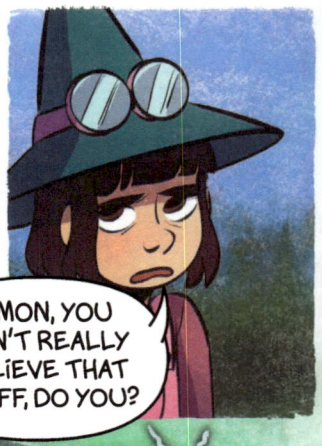

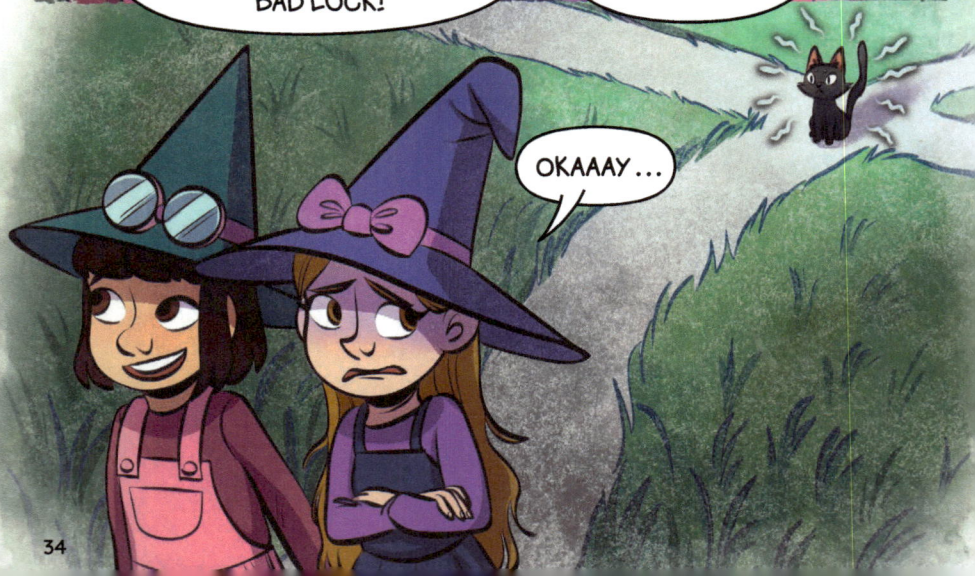

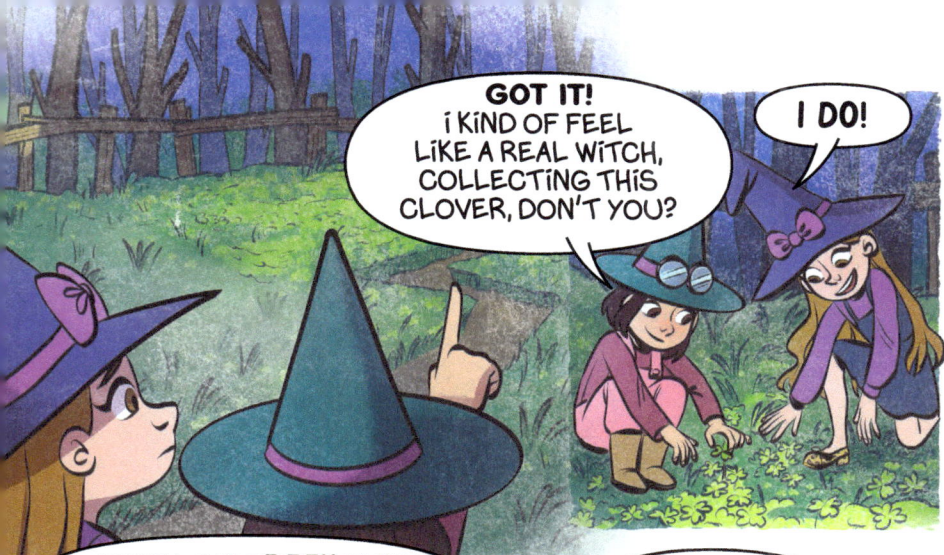

GOT IT! i KiND OF FEEL LIKE A REAL WITCH, COLLECTiNG THiS CLOVER, DON'T YOU?

I DO!

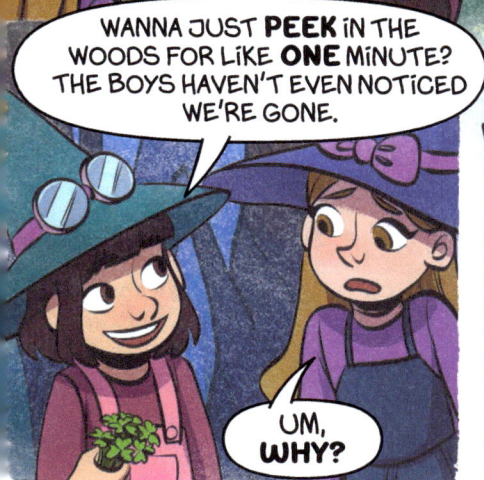

WANNA JUST PEEK iN THE WOODS FOR LiKE ONE MiNUTE? THE BOYS HAVEN'T EVEN NOTiCED WE'RE GONE.

UM, WHY?

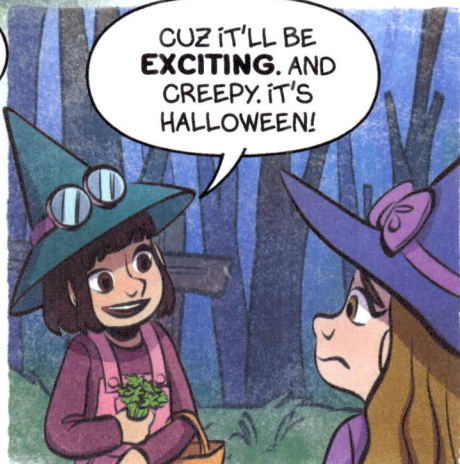

CUZ iT'LL BE EXCiTiNG. AND CREEPY. iT'S HALLOWEEN!

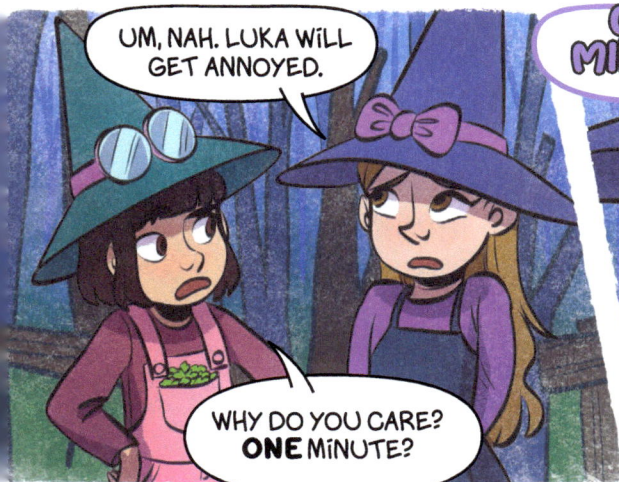

UM, NAH. LUKA WiLL GET ANNOYED.

WHY DO YOU CARE? ONE MiNUTE?

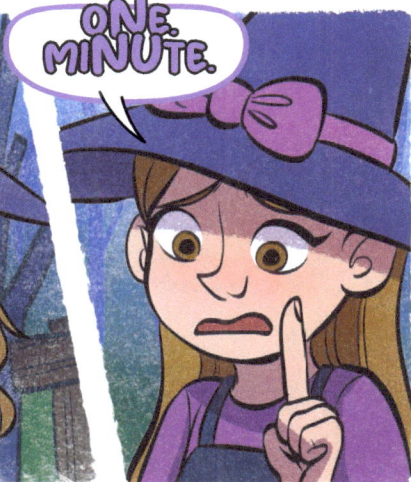

ONE MiNUTE.

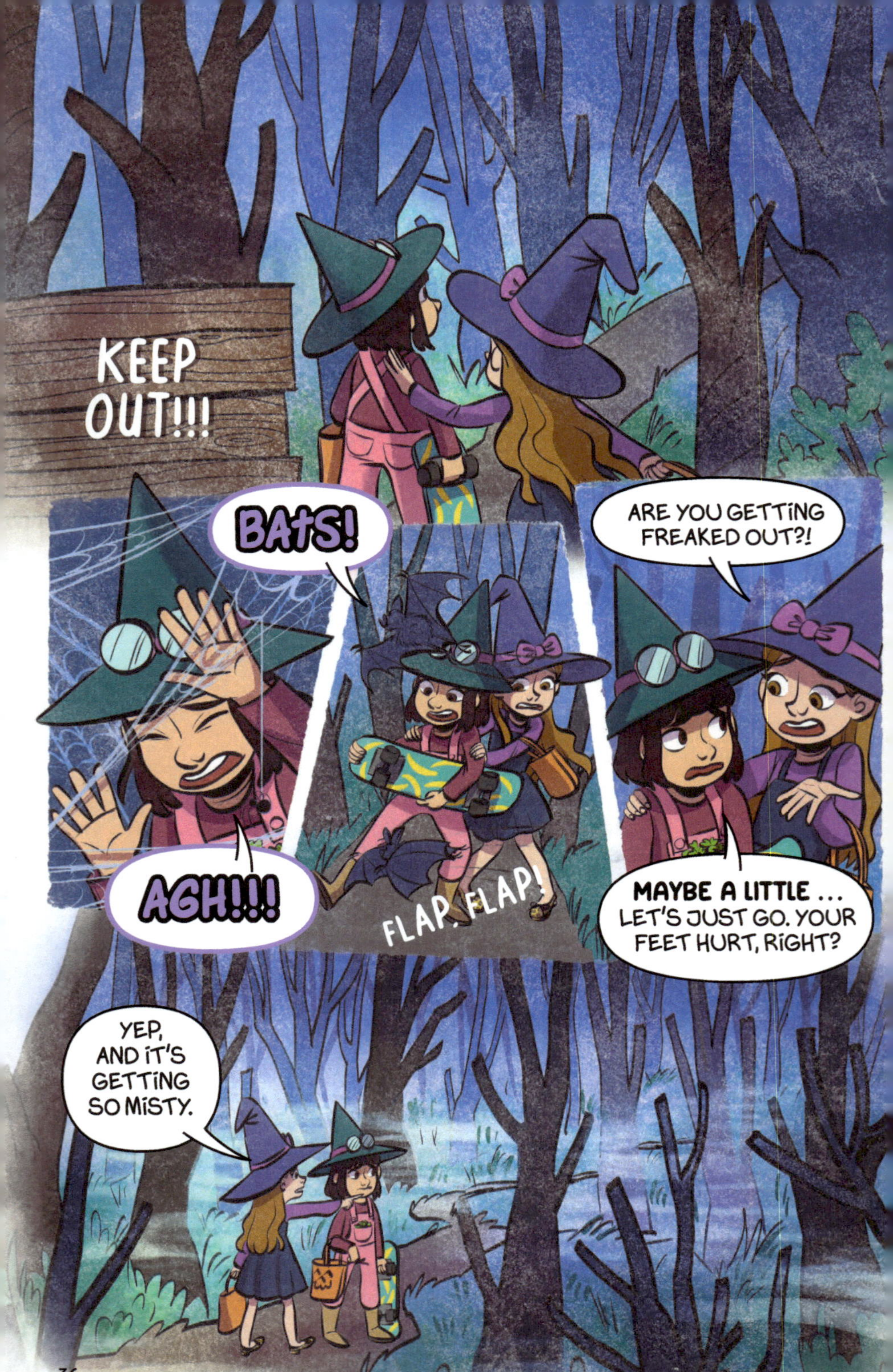
KEEP OUT!!!
AGH!!!
BATS!
FLAP, FLAP!
ARE YOU GETTING FREAKED OUT?!
MAYBE A LITTLE ... LET'S JUST GO. YOUR FEET HURT, RIGHT?
YEP, AND IT'S GETTING SO MISTY.

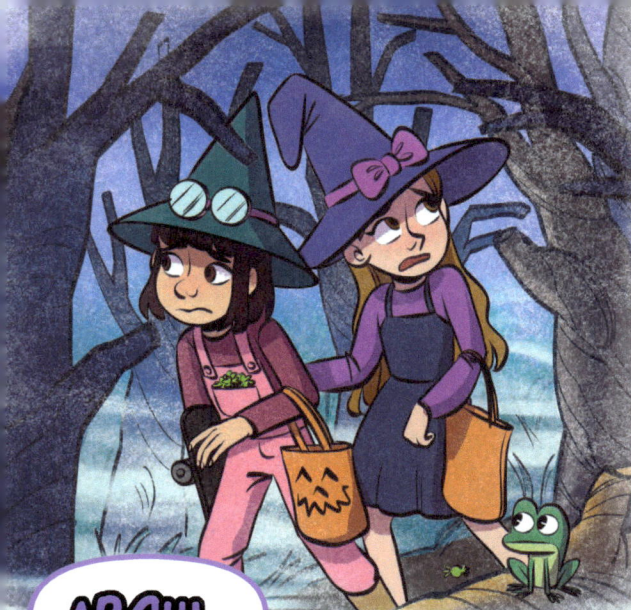

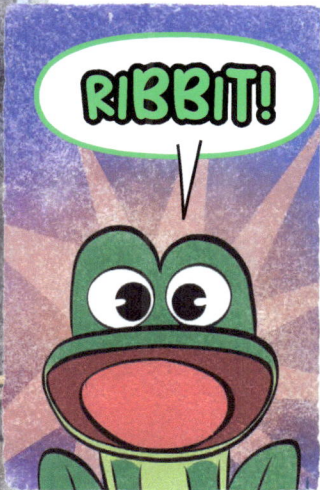

RIBBIT!

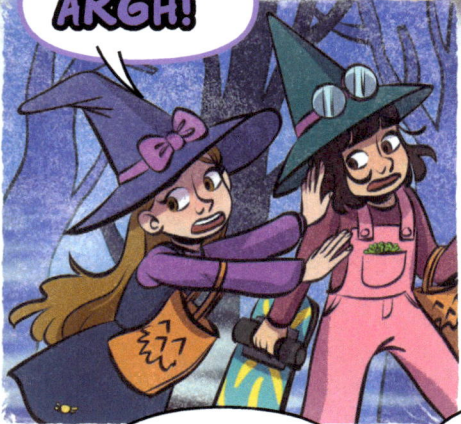

ARGH!

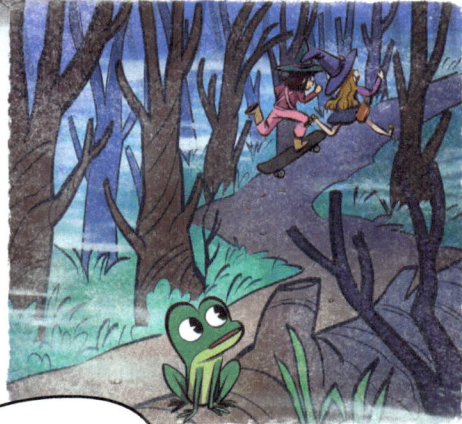

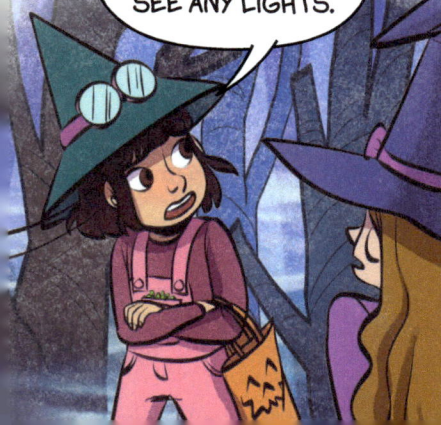

HEY. THIS WAY DOESN'T LOOK RIGHT. i CAN'T SEE ANY LIGHTS.

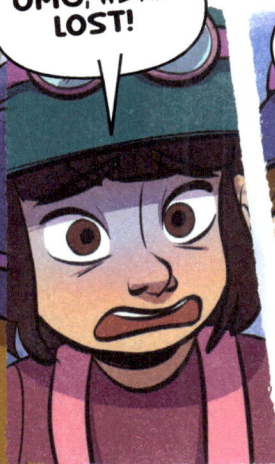

OMG, WE'RE LOST!

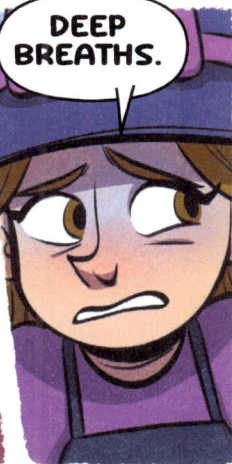

DEEP BREATHS.

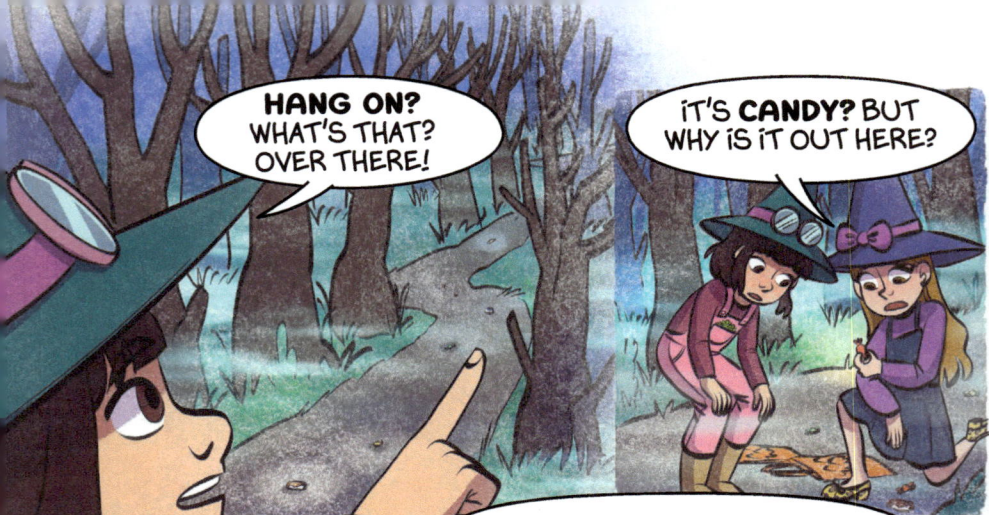

HANG ON? WHAT'S THAT? OVER THERE!

IT'S **CANDY?** BUT WHY IS IT OUT HERE?

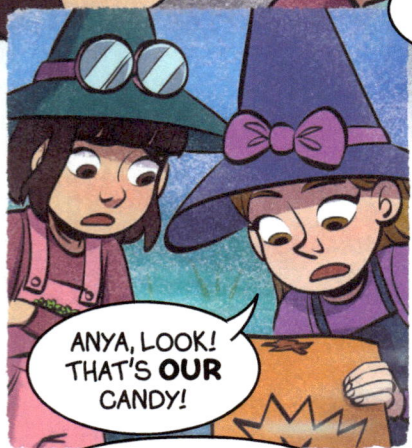

ANYA, LOOK! THAT'S **OUR** CANDY!

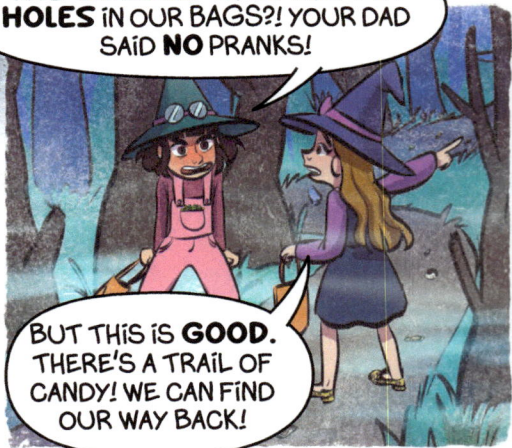

THE BOYS DID THIS!! THEY PUT **HOLES** IN OUR BAGS?! YOUR DAD SAID **NO** PRANKS!

BUT THIS IS **GOOD.** THERE'S A TRAIL OF CANDY! WE CAN FIND OUR WAY BACK!

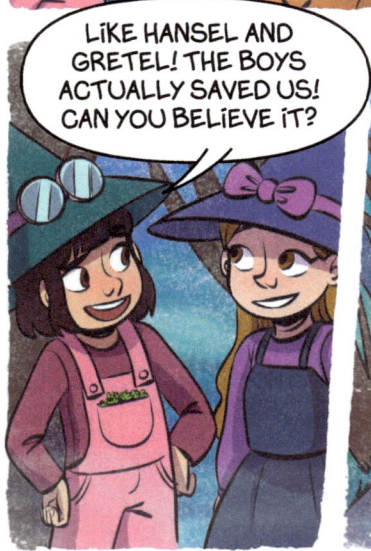

LIKE HANSEL AND GRETEL! THE BOYS ACTUALLY SAVED US! CAN YOU BELIEVE IT?

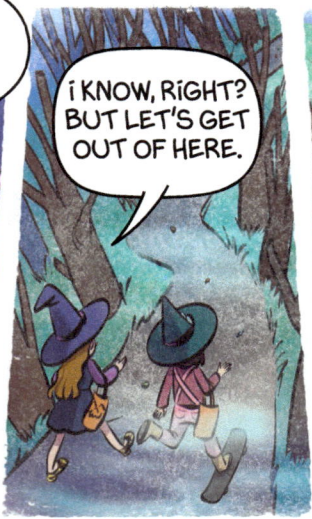

I KNOW, RIGHT? BUT LET'S GET OUT OF HERE.

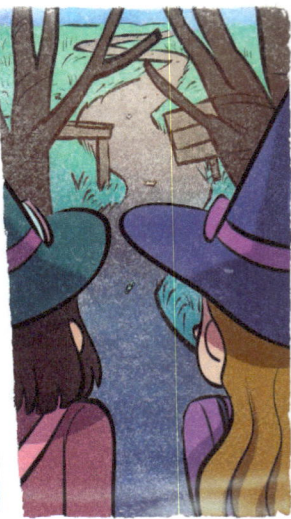

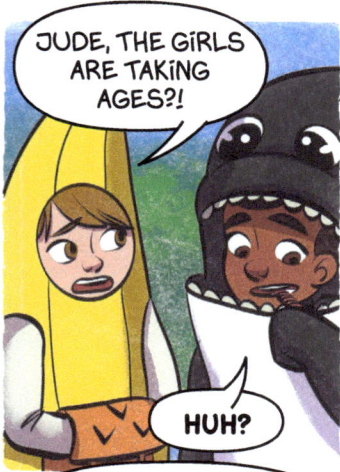

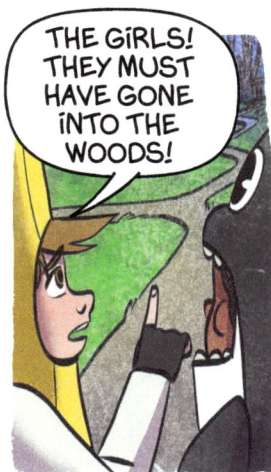

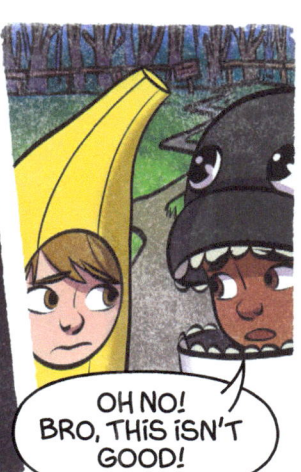

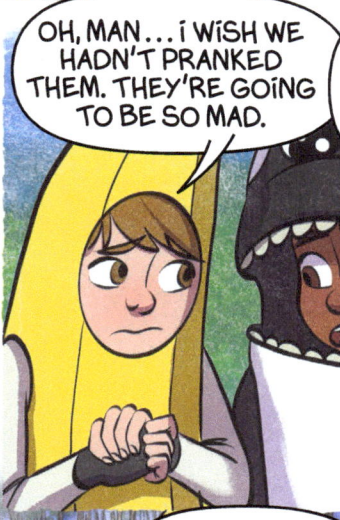

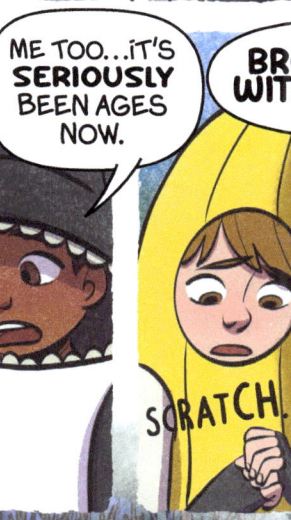

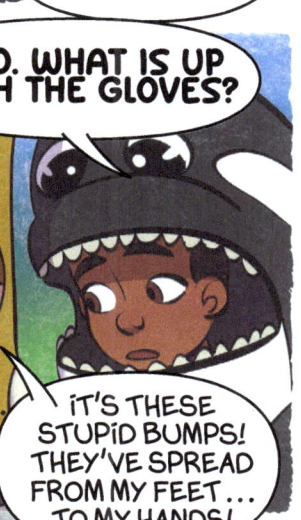

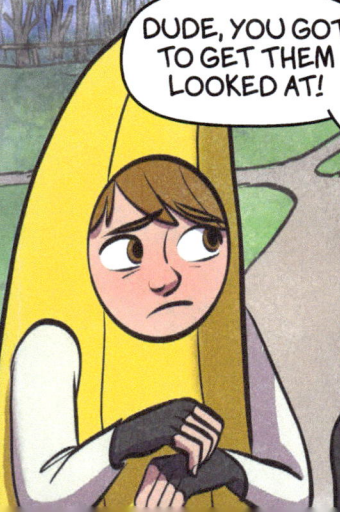

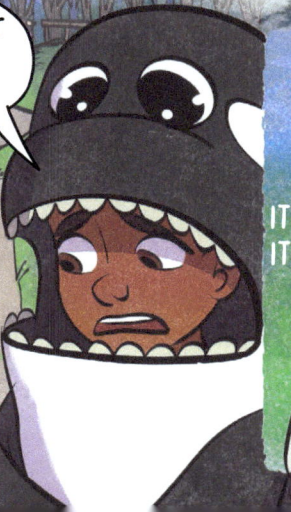

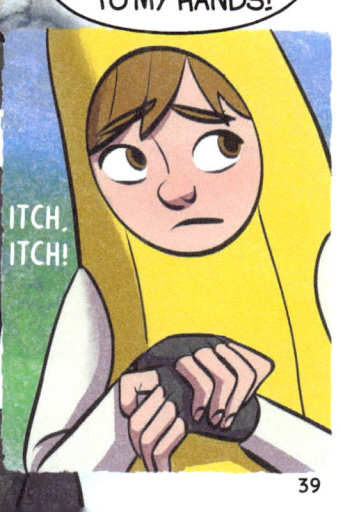

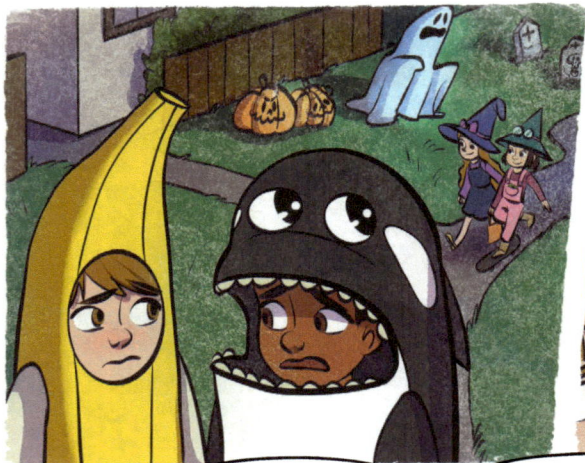

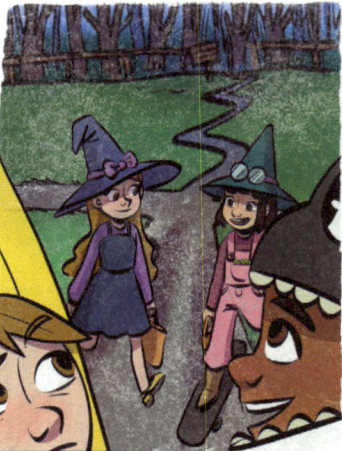

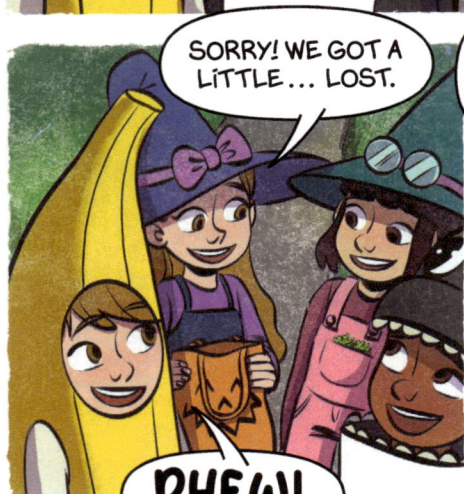

SORRY! WE GOT A LITTLE... LOST.

PHEW!

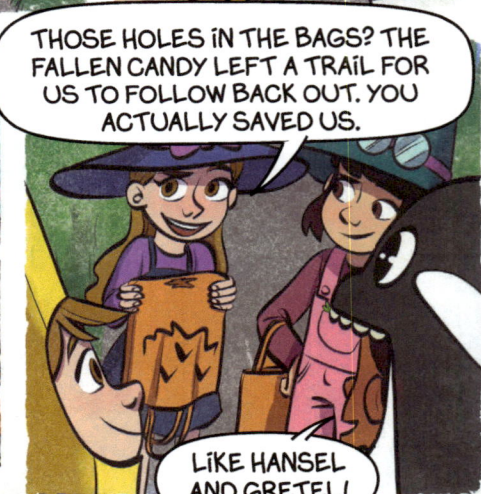

THOSE HOLES IN THE BAGS? THE FALLEN CANDY LEFT A TRAIL FOR US TO FOLLOW BACK OUT. YOU ACTUALLY SAVED US.

LIKE HANSEL AND GRETEL!

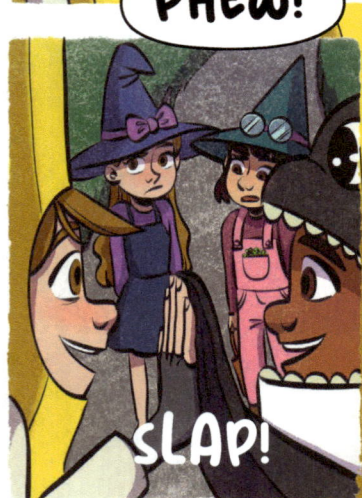

SLAP!

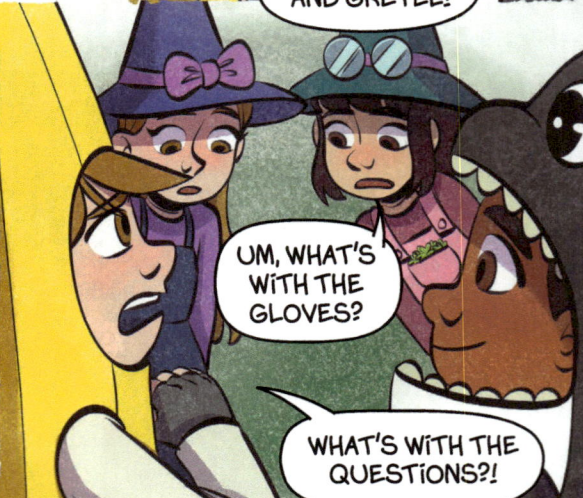

UM, WHAT'S WITH THE GLOVES?

WHAT'S WITH THE QUESTIONS?!

CHAPTER FOUR

Stir, bubble, pop, hiss!

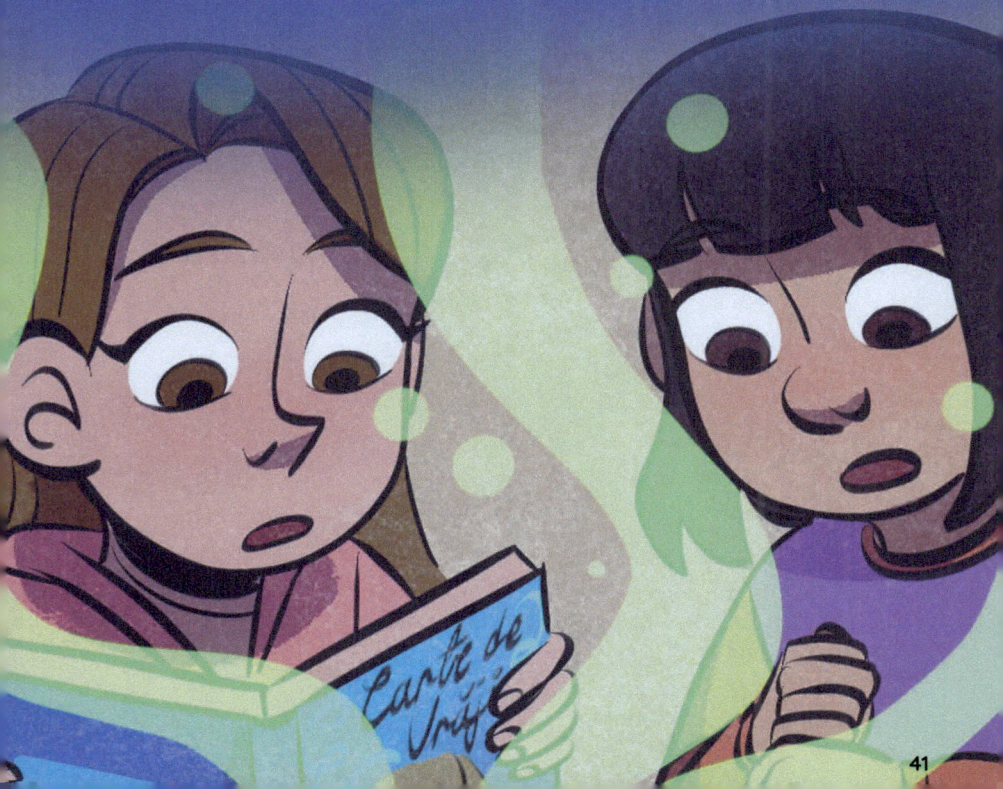

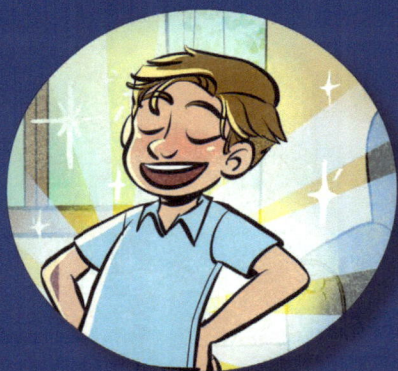

After all the drama, we went home and made the Halloween cookies...

Very special Halloween cookies... for Luka.

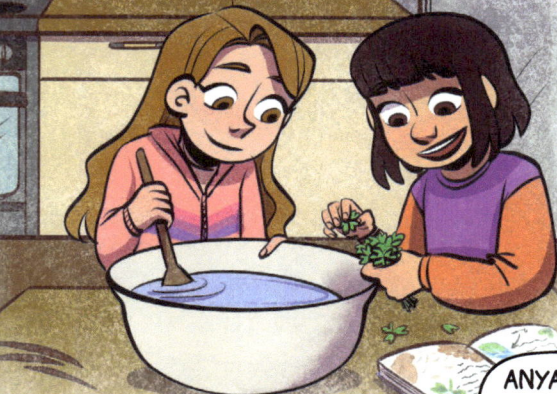

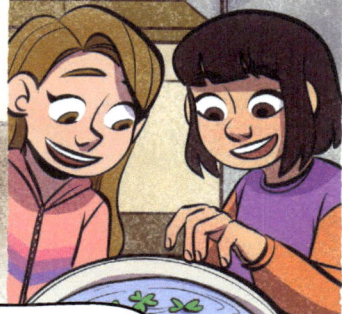

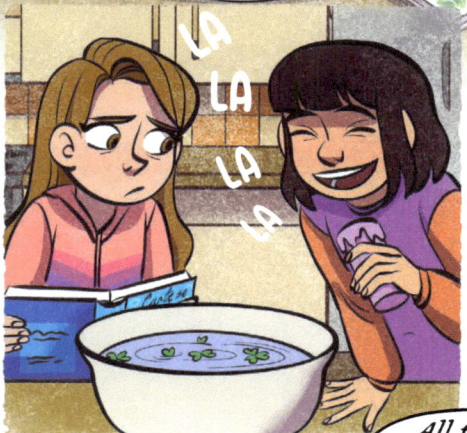

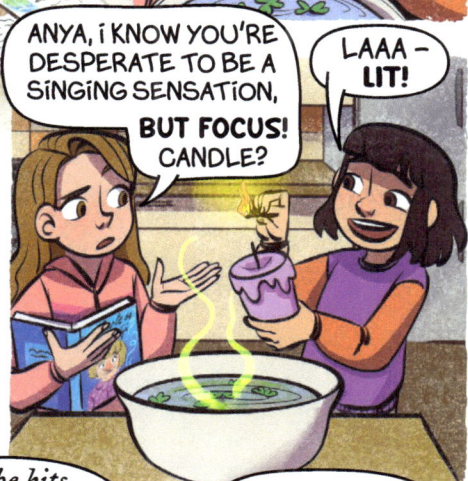

ANYA, I KNOW YOU'RE DESPERATE TO BE A SINGING SENSATION, **BUT FOCUS!** CANDLE?

LA LA LA LA

LAAA - **LIT!**

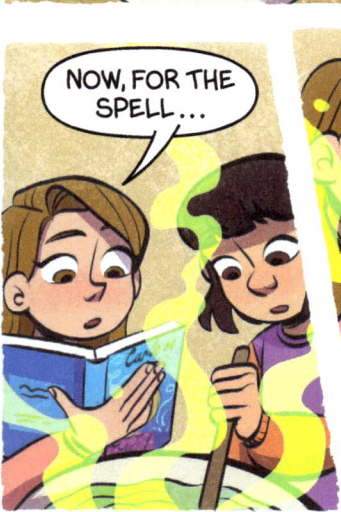

NOW, FOR THE SPELL...

All the bits Are in the pot, Will it work Or will it not?

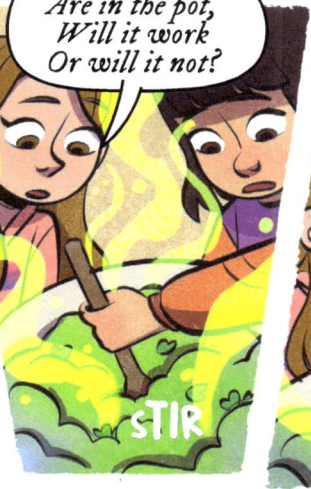

Make it bubble, Make it swell. Mix the potion, Mix it well.

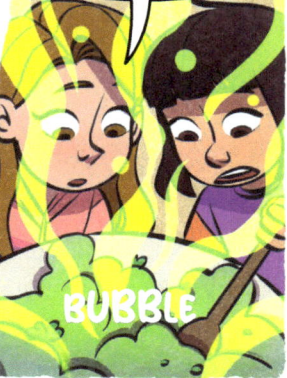

STIR

BUBBLE

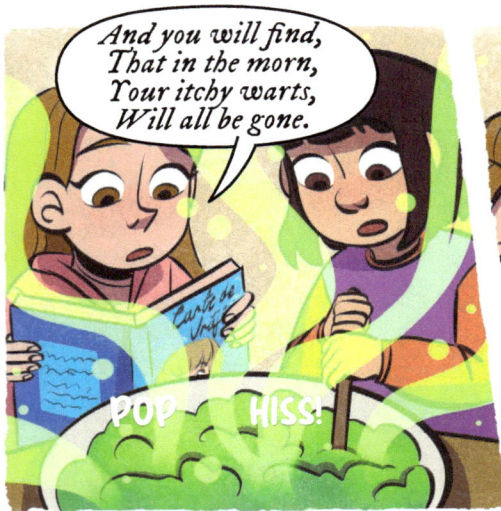

And you will find,
That in the morn,
Your itchy warts,
Will all be gone.

POP HISS!

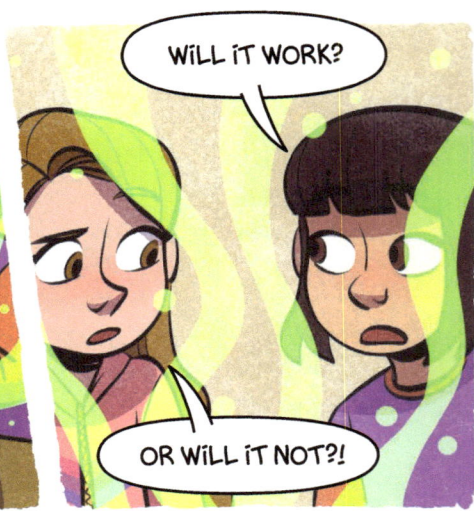

WILL IT WORK?

OR WILL IT NOT?!

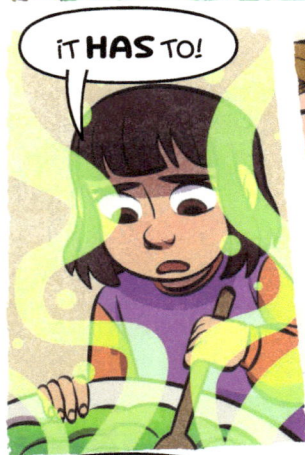

IT **HAS** TO!

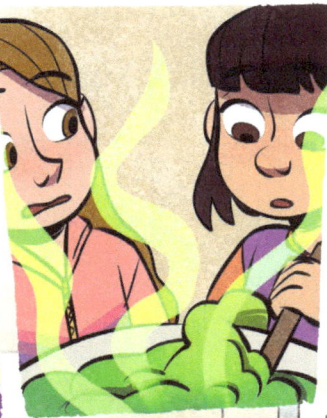

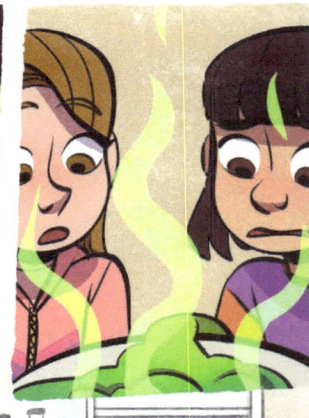

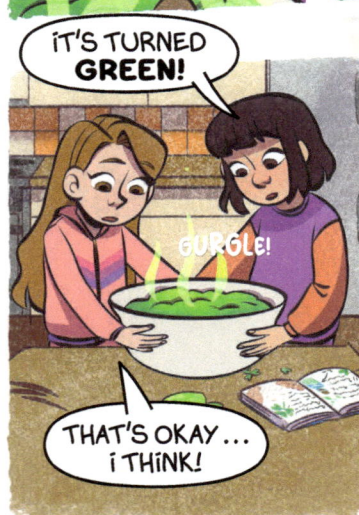

IT'S TURNED **GREEN!**

GURGLE!

THAT'S OKAY ... I THINK!

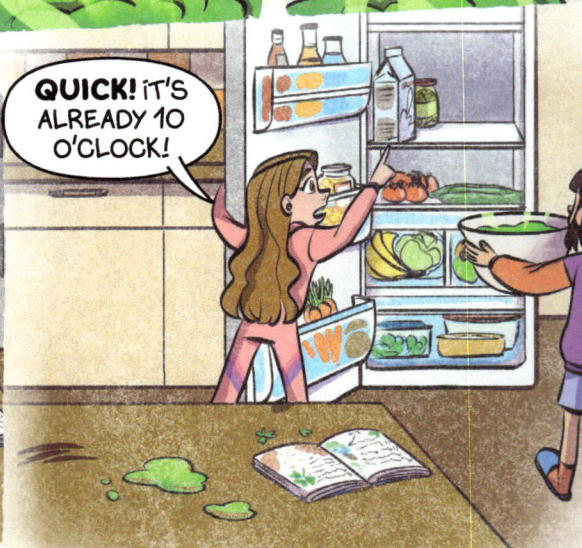

QUICK! IT'S ALREADY 10 O'CLOCK!

We waited for the potion to cool down...

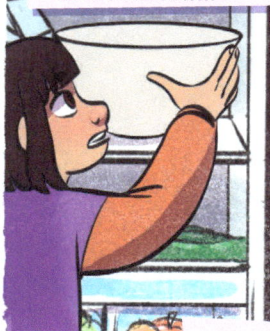

...stirred it into the cookie dough...

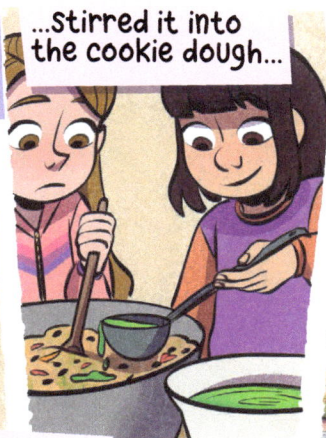

...and put it straight into the oven.

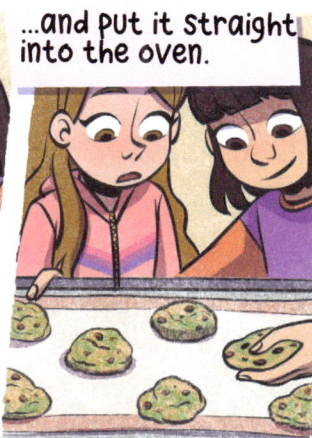

And when they were ready...

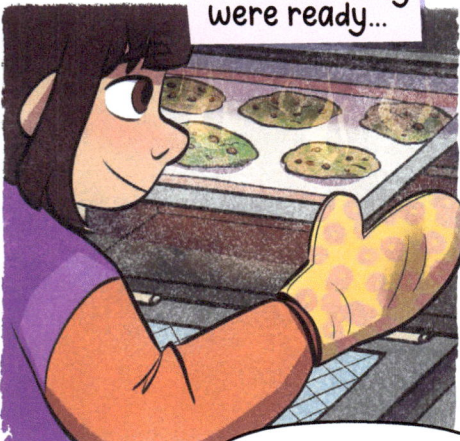

LUKA! HAVE A COOKIE! i KNOW YOU **LOVE** A LATE–NiGHT SNACK!

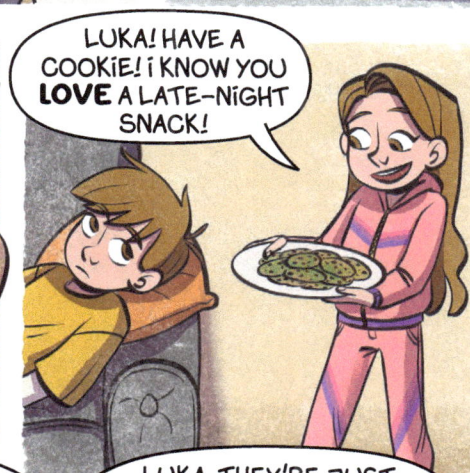

GREEN COOKiES?! OH, UM, i THiNK i'M OKAY.

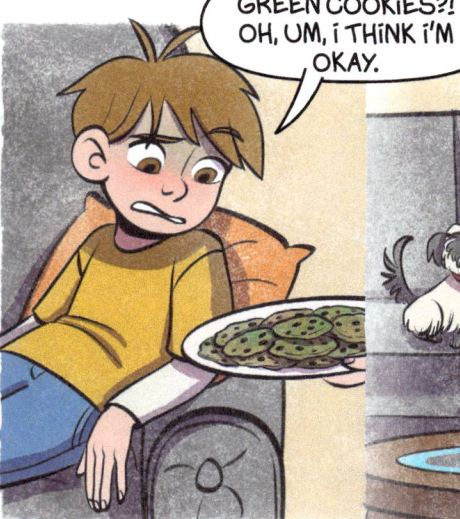

LUKA, THEY'RE JUST GREEN FOR HALLOWEEN! DON'T BE SO SCARED OF NEW THiNGS!

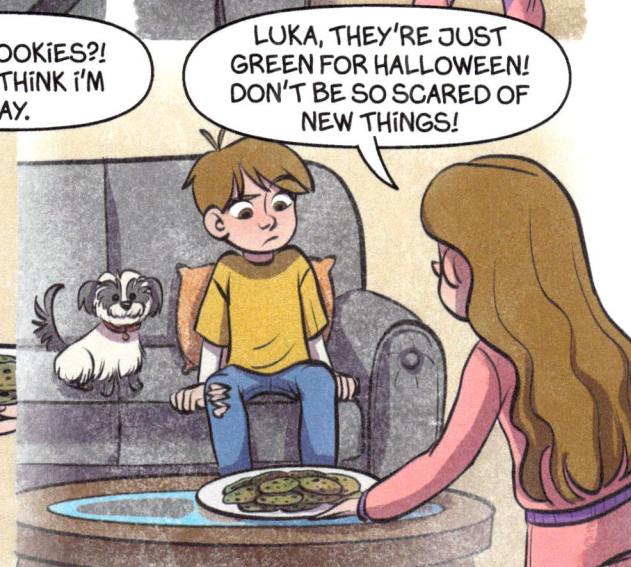

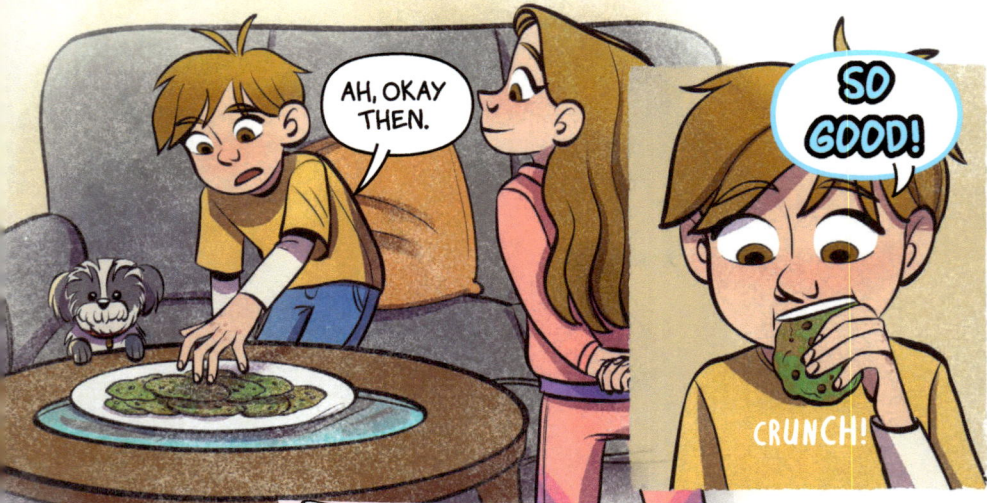

Then the potion got to work! well, we hoped it did.

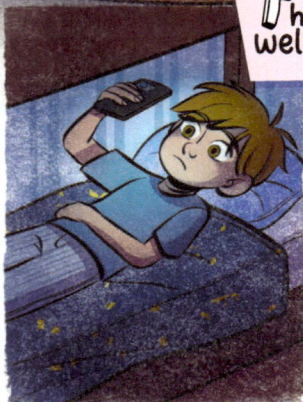
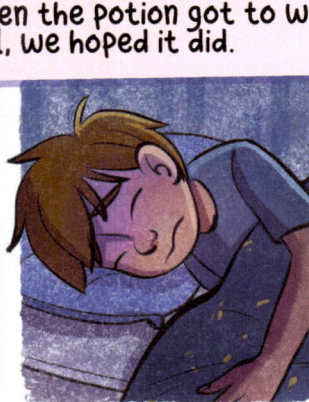
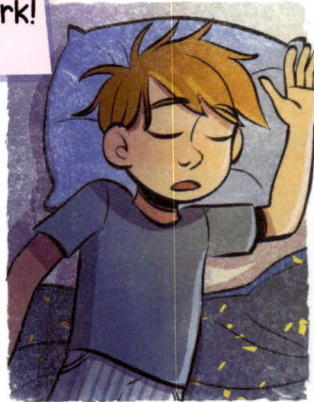

THE NEXT DAY...

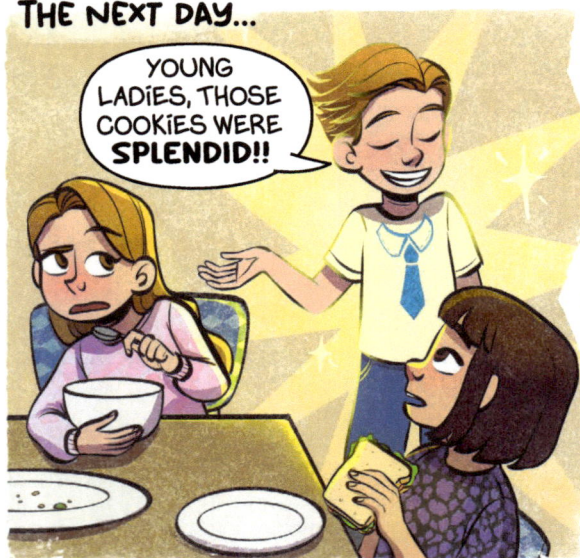

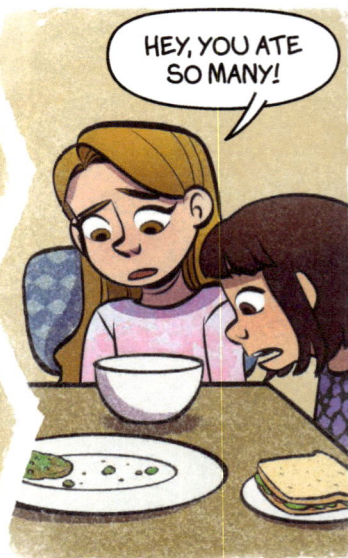

TAP TAP

SCRATCH

SCRATCH

SCRATCH

SCRATCH

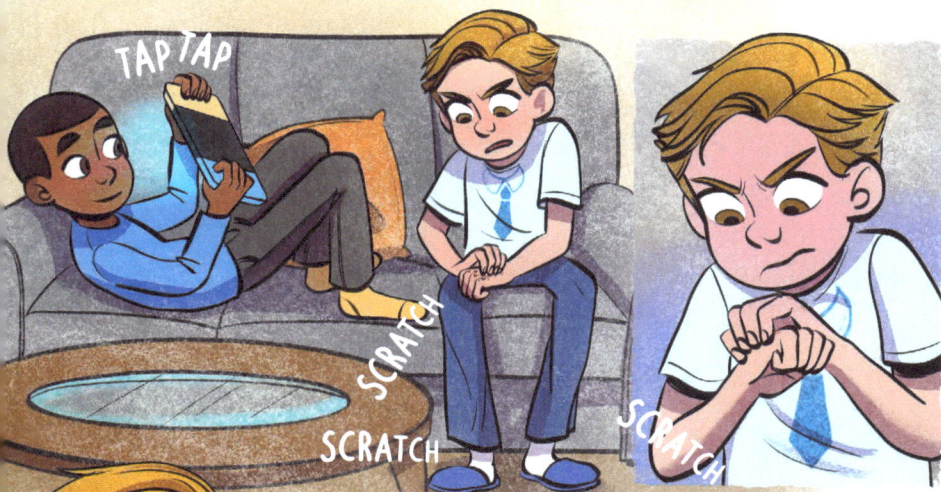

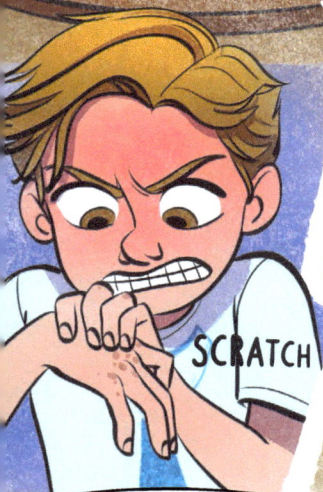

ANYA, HE'S STILL SCRATCHING! THE POTION DIDN'T WORK!

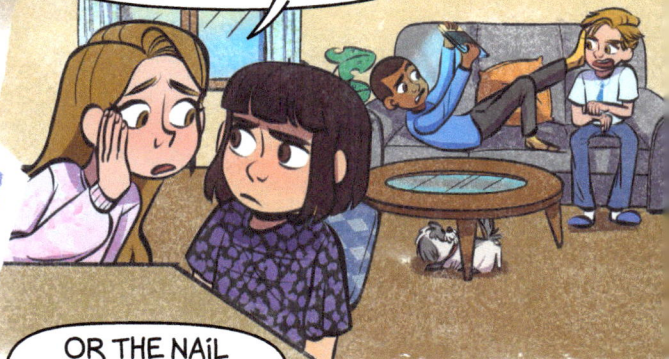

MUST HAVE BEEN THE PURPLE CANDLE.

OR THE NAIL POLISH ON OUR TOENAILS.

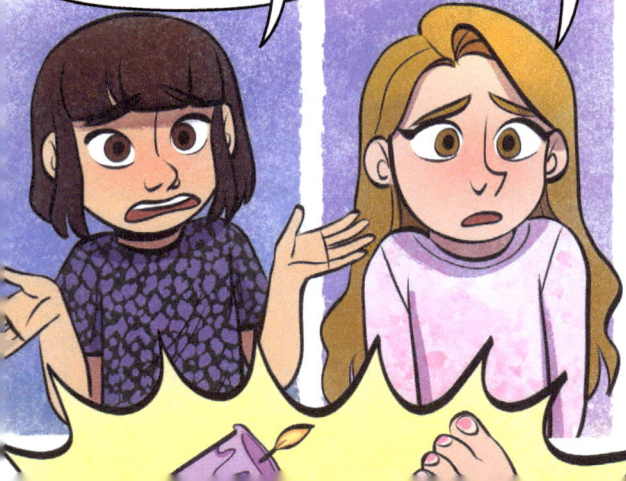

YEAH, NO CHANGE AT ALL IN THE WARTS!

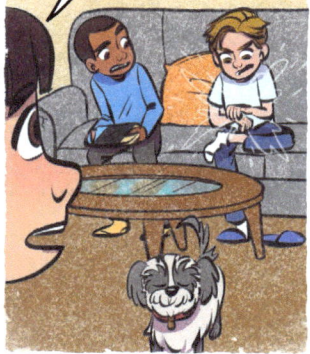

BRO. YOU'RE DRIVING ME CRAZY WITH ALL THAT **SCRATCHING!** YOU GOTTA SEE **DR. ITCH!**

BUT THEN WE'LL HAVE TO LEAVE **AND** DR. ITCH WILL THINK I'M **ABSOLUTELY HIDEOUS!**

DUDE, YOU'RE NOT HIDEOUS. YOU'RE **ANNOYING!**

I THINK YOU NEED TO TAKE LUKA TO SEE DR. ITCH. HIS ITCHING IS DRIVING **ME,** I MEAN, HIM, CRAZY.

MR. DAD!

NOW, LET ME FIND HER NUMBER...

IS THAT SO? YOU MEAN DR. LAZIC? HMM. I THINKS THAT'S A **WONDERFUL** IDEA, A **SENSIBLE** IDEA IS WHAT I AM TRYING TO SAY.

WHAT IS IT, BUDDY?

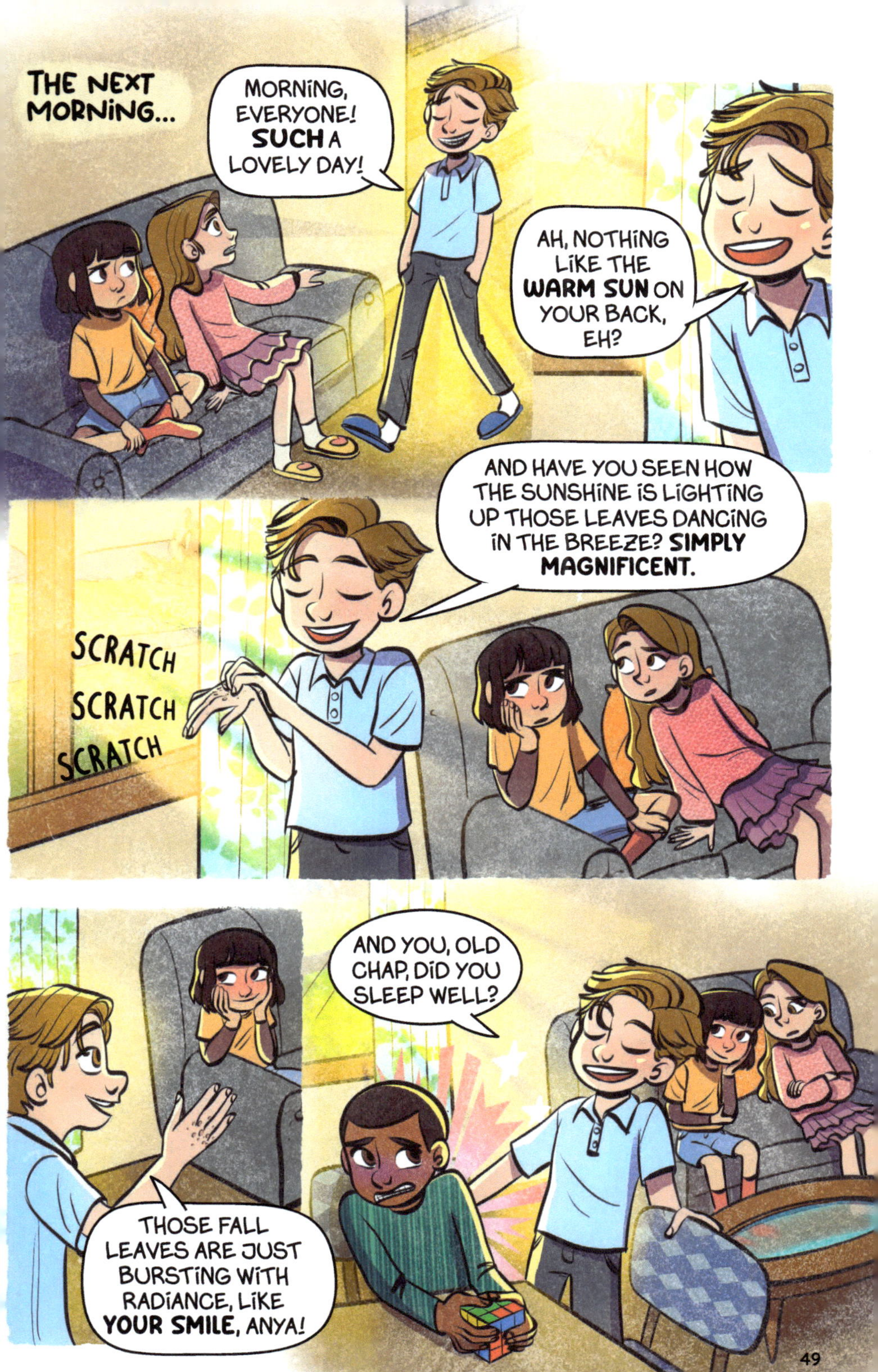
THE NEXT MORNING...
MORNING, EVERYONE! SUCH A LOVELY DAY!
AH, NOTHING LIKE THE WARM SUN ON YOUR BACK, EH?
AND HAVE YOU SEEN HOW THE SUNSHINE IS LIGHTING UP THOSE LEAVES DANCING IN THE BREEZE? SIMPLY MAGNIFICENT.
SCRATCH
SCRATCH
SCRATCH
THOSE FALL LEAVES ARE JUST BURSTING WITH RADIANCE, LIKE YOUR SMILE, ANYA!
AND YOU, OLD CHAP, DID YOU SLEEP WELL?

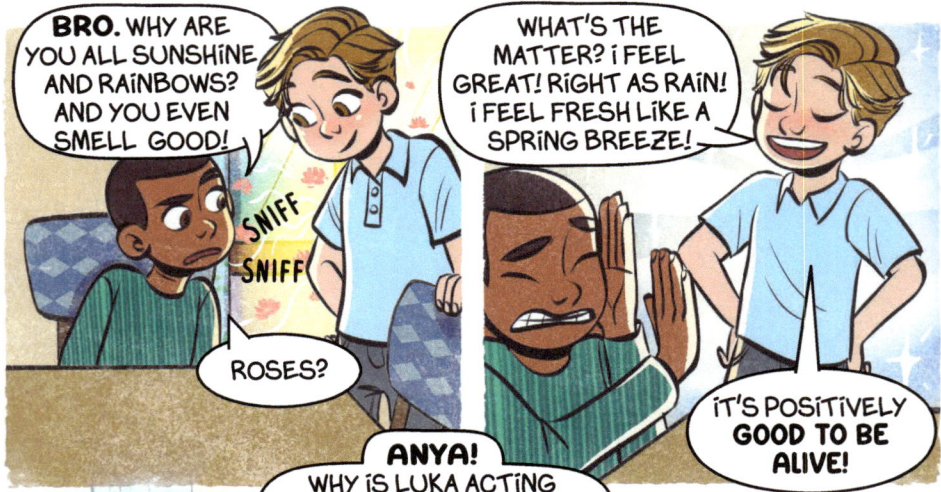

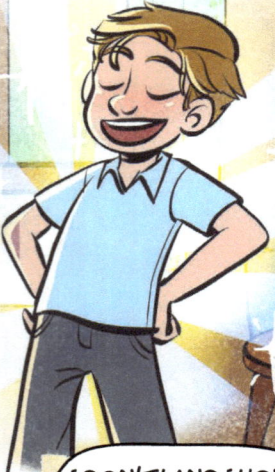

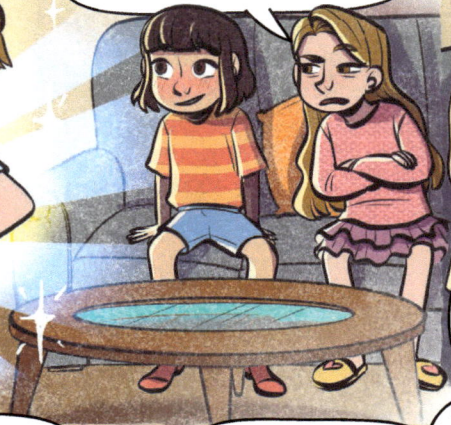

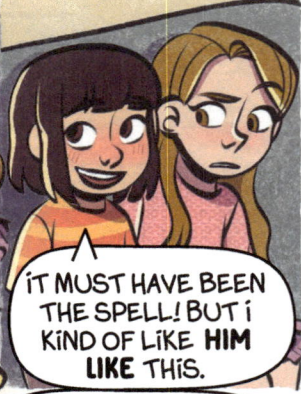

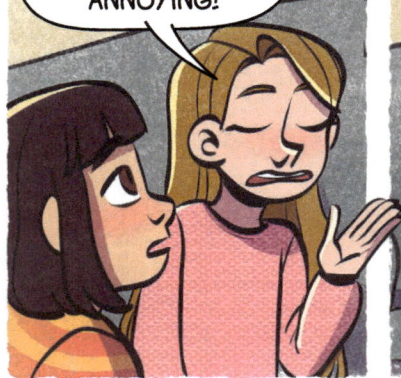

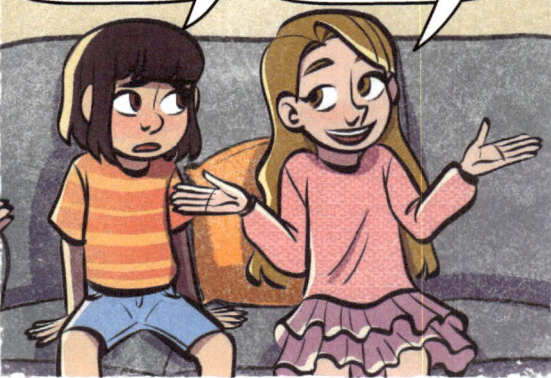

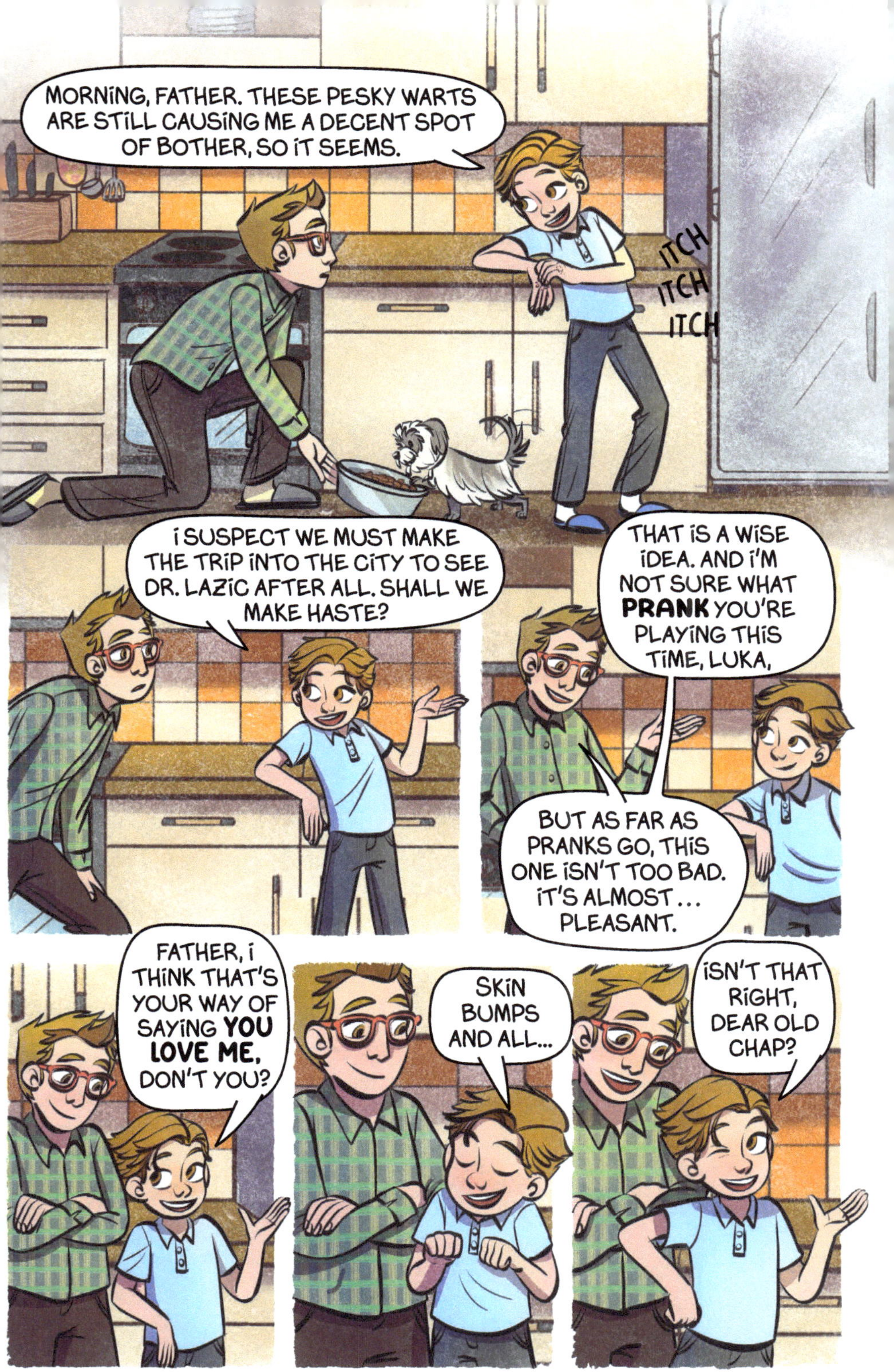
MORNING, FATHER. THESE PESKY WARTS ARE STILL CAUSING ME A DECENT SPOT OF BOTHER, SO IT SEEMS.
ITCH ITCH ITCH
I SUSPECT WE MUST MAKE THE TRIP INTO THE CITY TO SEE DR. LAZIC AFTER ALL. SHALL WE MAKE HASTE?
THAT IS A WISE IDEA. AND I'M NOT SURE WHAT **PRANK** YOU'RE PLAYING THIS TIME, LUKA,
BUT AS FAR AS PRANKS GO, THIS ONE ISN'T TOO BAD. IT'S ALMOST . . . PLEASANT.
FATHER, I THINK THAT'S YOUR WAY OF SAYING **YOU LOVE ME,** DON'T YOU?
SKIN BUMPS AND ALL...
ISN'T THAT RIGHT, DEAR OLD CHAP?

OF COURSE I DO.

LET'S **GO**, YOU SILLY KIDDOS!!

OKAY, TIDDLY-HO, OFF WE GO!

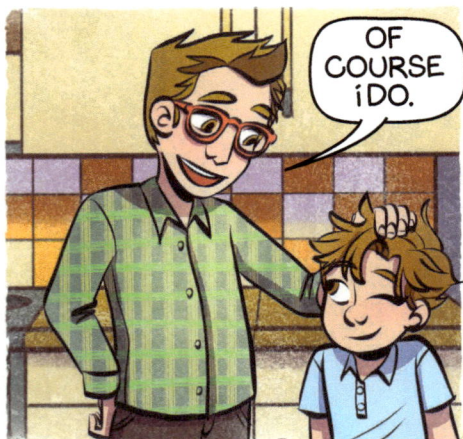

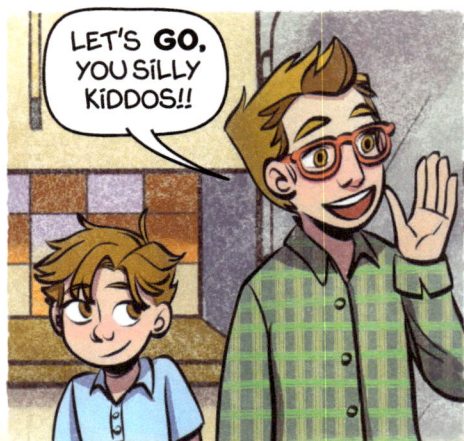

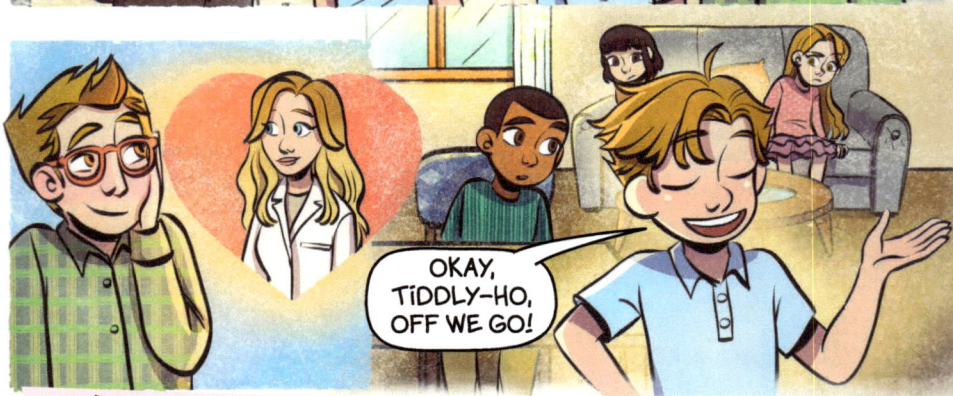

We packed up and headed back to the city. So bummed to leave early!

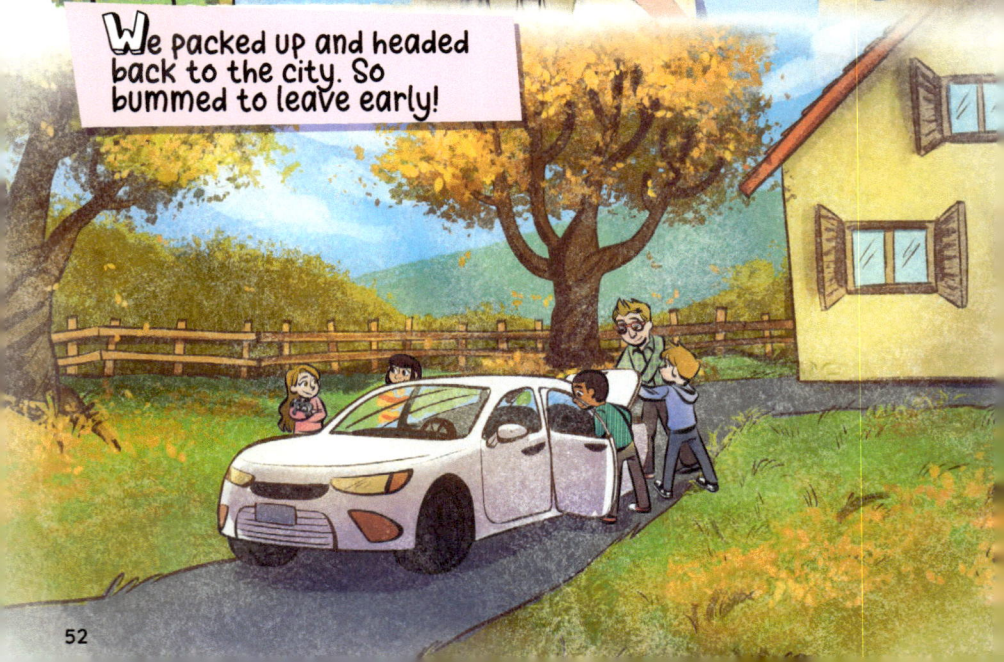

CHAPTER FIVE

Beetle Juice!

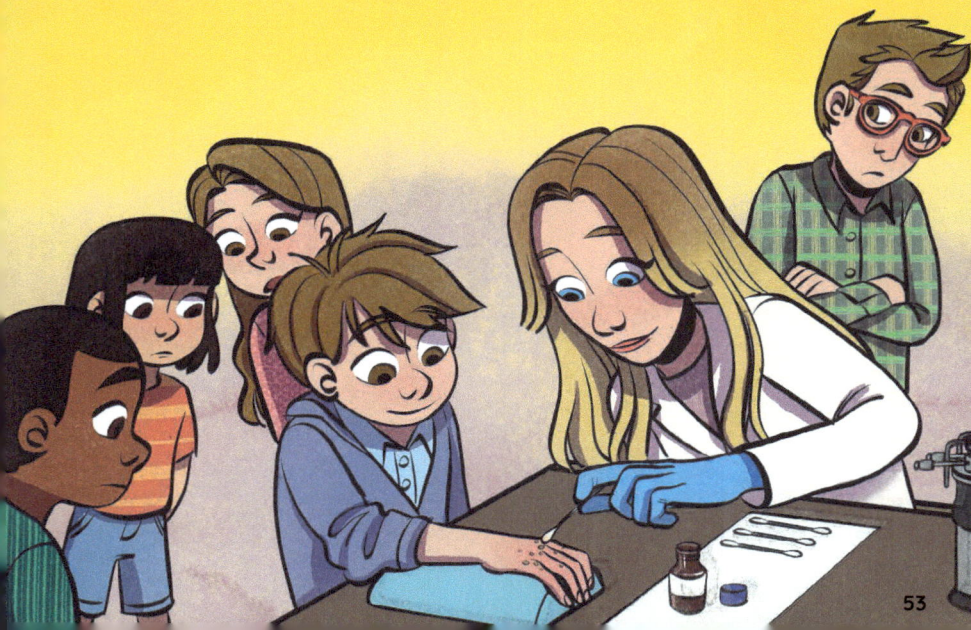

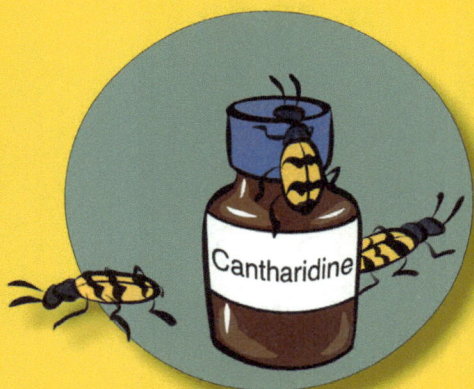

WELCOME! My name is Cutis. Let me take you to Dr. Lazic. Follow me.

DAD, YOU GOTTA ASK DR. iTCH ON A **DATE** THIS TIME. WE ALL KNOW YOU **LIKE** HER.

A D-D-DATE? UM, SHOULD i? YOU THINK SHE'D **SAY YES???**

YEAH, SHE WiLL!

WELL, ALRIGHT, iF YOU REALLY THINK SO?

i DO! PiNKY PROMISE?

DID YOU KNOW THAT ORCAS SLEEP...

...WITH ONE EYE OPEN!

YEAH, THAT'S RIGHT! AND THE REASON IS NOT TO KEEP AN EYE OUT FOR **PREDATORS** BUT...

...TO CONTROL THEIR BREATHING!

YES! HEY, THERE'S THIS COOL WHALE EXHIBIT NEXT MONTH. **WANNA COME?**

SURE, I THINK I CAN FIND SOME TIME IN MY SCHEDULE.

HI GUYS!

HI DR. ITCH, I MEAN, DR. LAZIC!

YOU CAN CALL ME **DR. ITCH.**

NOW, HOW CAN I HELP TODAY?

LUKA HERE HAS SOME ITCHY **BUMPS** ON HIS FOOT THAT HAVE SPREAD TO HIS HANDS.

OH, NOTHING TO BE EMBARRASSED ABOUT.

I HAVE KIDS IN HERE ALL THE TIME WITH JUST THE SAME KIND OF BUMPS. LET ME **TAKE A LOOK.**

THANK YOU KINDLY, DR. LAZIC. I AM SO **VERY GRATEFUL** FOR YOUR SERVICES.

SURE, MY PLEASURE.

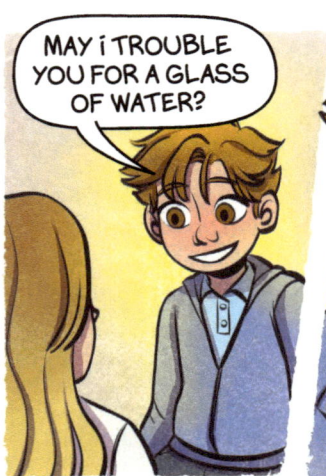

MAY I TROUBLE YOU FOR A GLASS OF WATER?

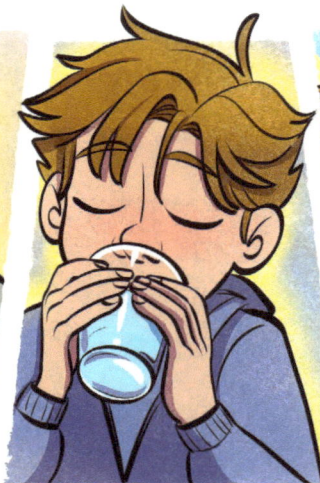

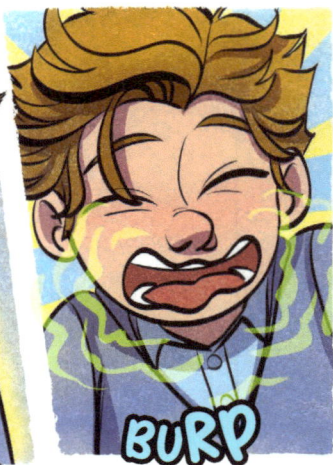

BURP

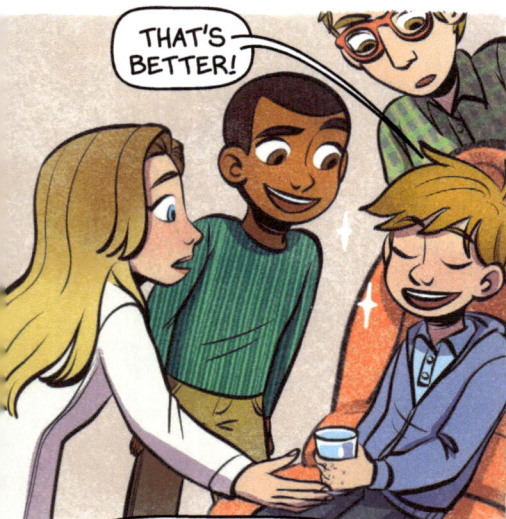

THAT'S BETTER!

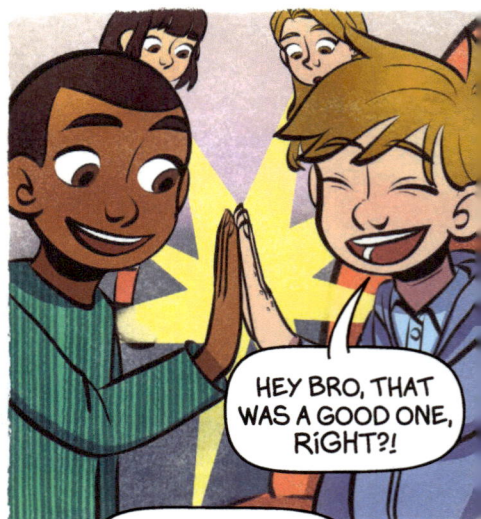

HEY BRO, THAT WAS A GOOD ONE, RIGHT?!

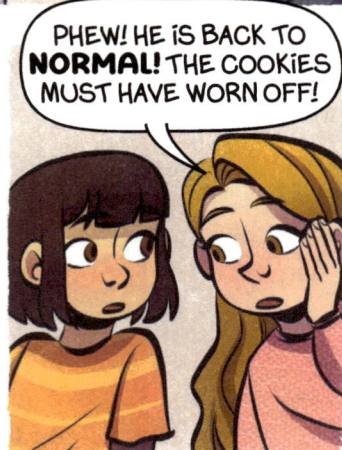

PHEW! HE IS BACK TO **NORMAL!** THE COOKIES MUST HAVE WORN OFF!

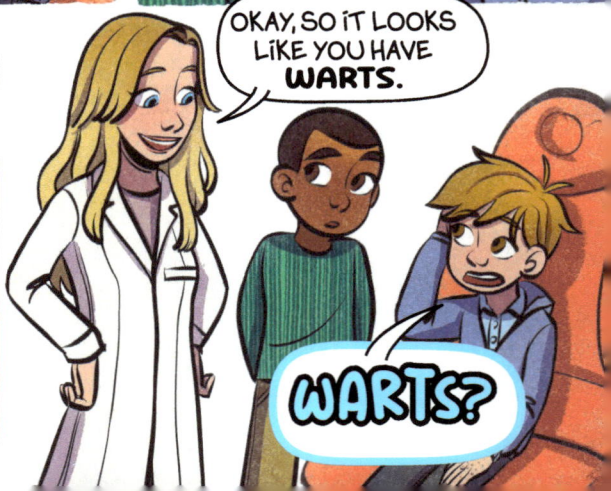

OKAY, SO IT LOOKS LIKE YOU HAVE **WARTS.**

WARTS?

WARTS ARE QUITE COMMON, A BIT STUBBORN BUT VERY TREATABLE.

BUT I DIDN'T TOUCH A **TOAD!**

WELL, THEY ACTUALLY SPREAD FROM PERSON TO PERSON.

They are caused by a virus called HPV, the HUMAN PAPILLOMAVIRUS.

And can be found on any part of the body.

YOU CAN CATCH IT IF, SAY, YOU WALK **BAREFOOT** AT A PUBLIC POOL OR PUBLIC SHOWER, OR...

LUKA! DID YOU WEAR FLIP-FLOPS IN THE SHOWER AT SUMMER CAMP?!

UH, NO, I DIDN'T.

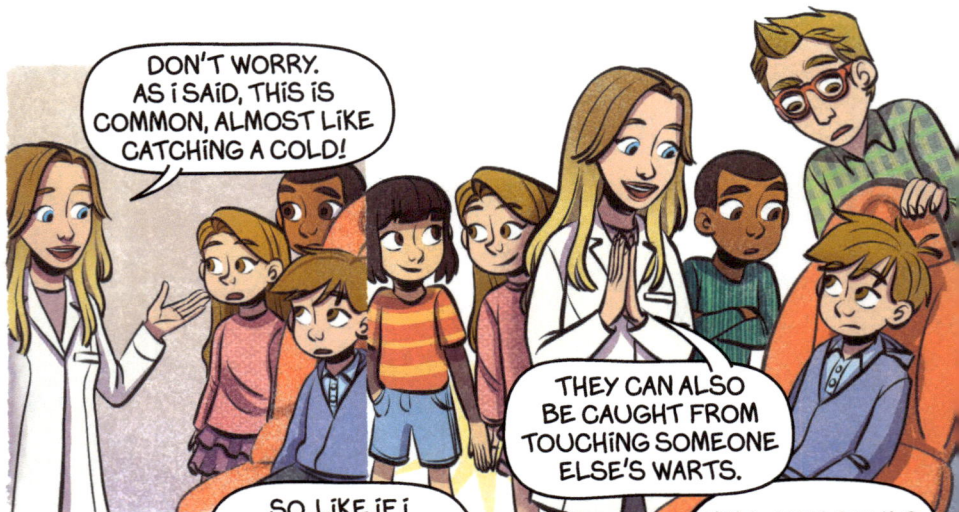

DON'T WORRY. AS I SAID, THIS IS COMMON, ALMOST LIKE CATCHING A COLD!

THEY CAN ALSO BE CAUGHT FROM TOUCHING SOMEONE ELSE'S WARTS.

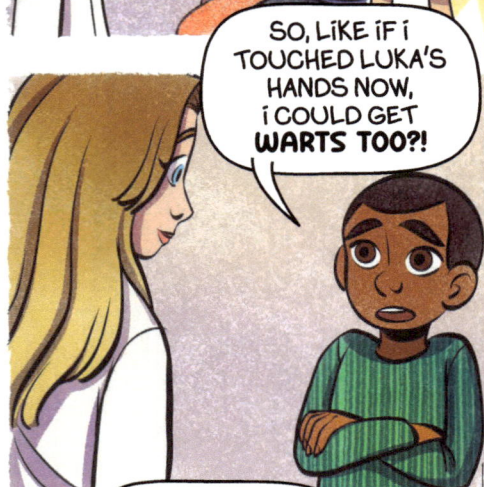

SO, LIKE IF I TOUCHED LUKA'S HANDS NOW, I COULD GET **WARTS TOO?!**

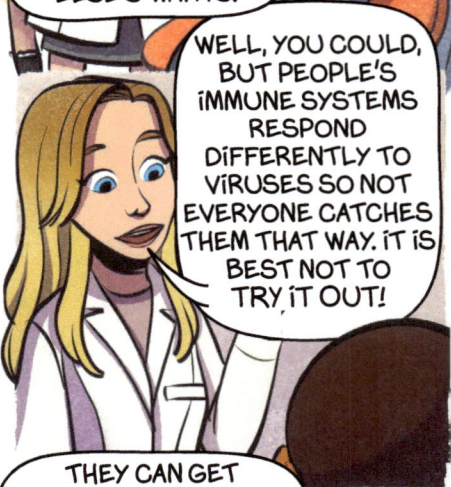

WELL, YOU COULD, BUT PEOPLE'S IMMUNE SYSTEMS RESPOND DIFFERENTLY TO VIRUSES SO NOT EVERYONE CATCHES THEM THAT WAY. IT IS BEST NOT TO TRY IT OUT!

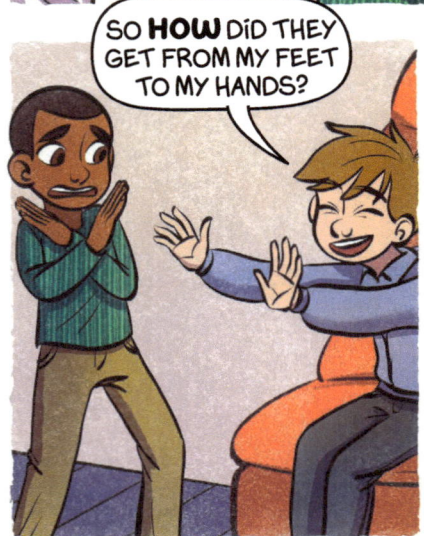

SO **HOW** DID THEY GET FROM MY FEET TO MY HANDS?

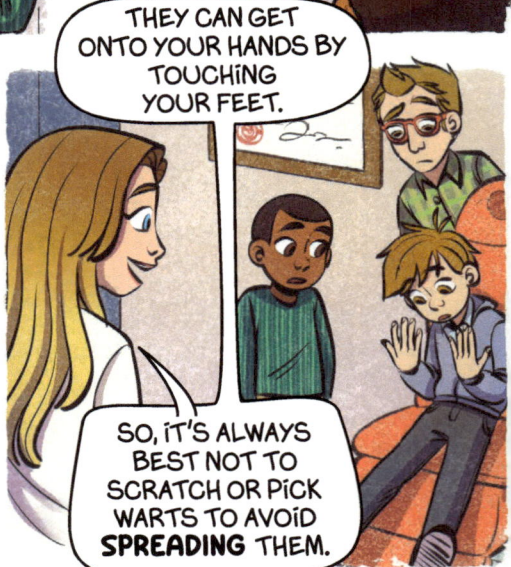

THEY CAN GET ONTO YOUR HANDS BY TOUCHING YOUR FEET.

SO, IT'S ALWAYS BEST NOT TO SCRATCH OR PICK WARTS TO AVOID **SPREADING** THEM.

YOU WERE SCRATCHING LIKE **CRAZY**, DUDE.

AH, SO IF LIKE I, I MEAN, IF LUKA PICKED HIS NOSE, HE COULD GET THEM IN HIS **NOSE AND FACE?!**

YES, HE COULD.

BETTER STOP PICKING YOUR NOSE, BRO!

SO, IS THAT WHY **WITCHES** HAVE WARTS ON **THEIR NOSES?!** THEY PICK THEM?!

WELL, THAT'S VERY POSSIBLE! BUT THOSE ARE PROBABLY MOLES.

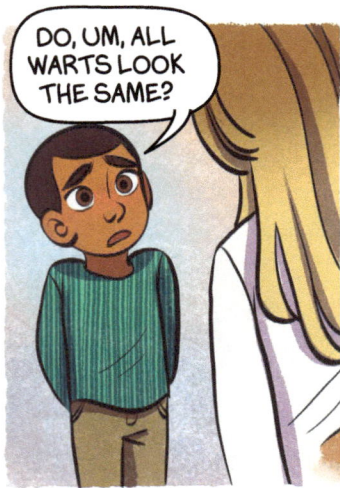

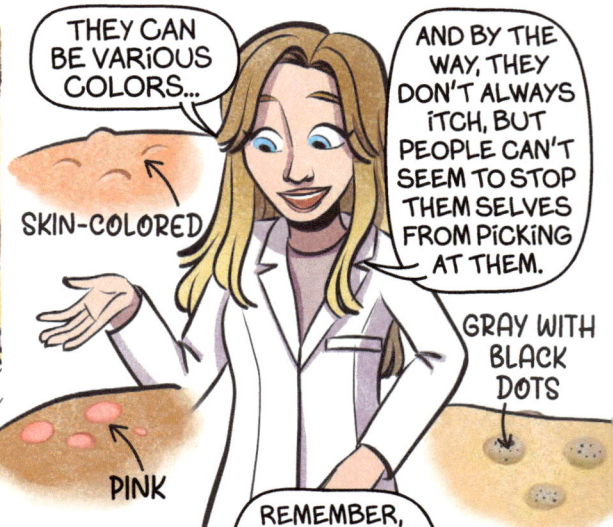

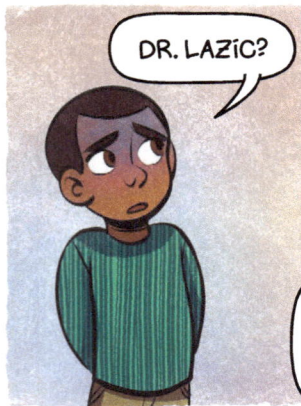

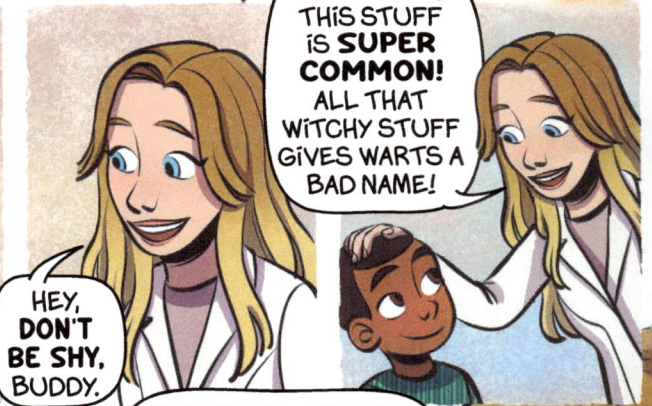

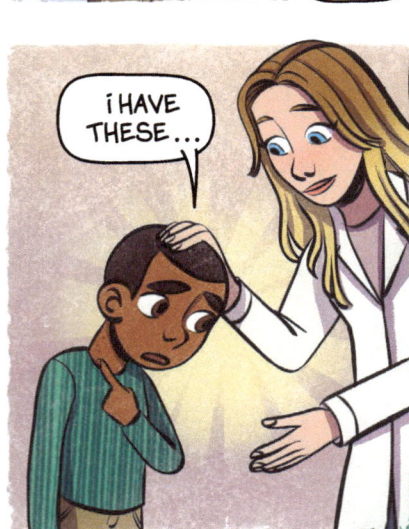

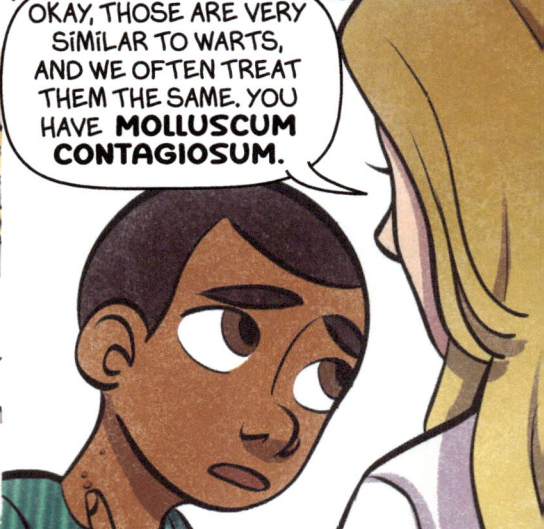

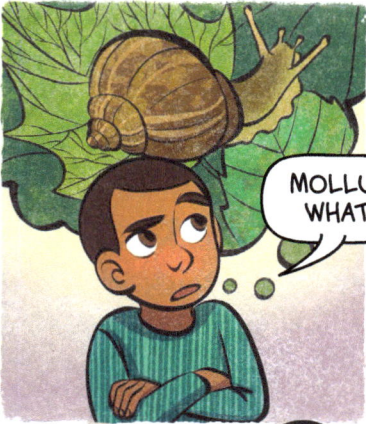

MOLLUSC WHAT??

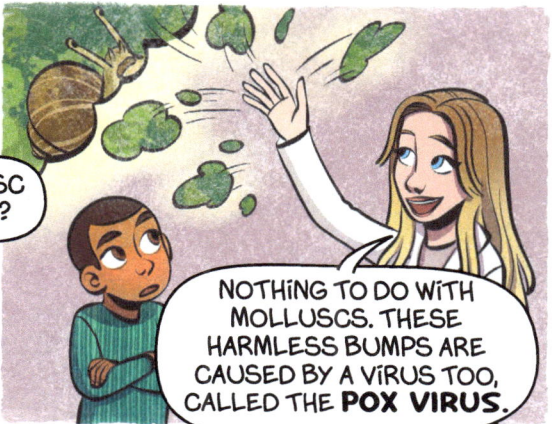

NOTHING TO DO WITH MOLLUSCS. THESE HARMLESS BUMPS ARE CAUSED BY A VIRUS TOO, CALLED THE **POX VIRUS**.

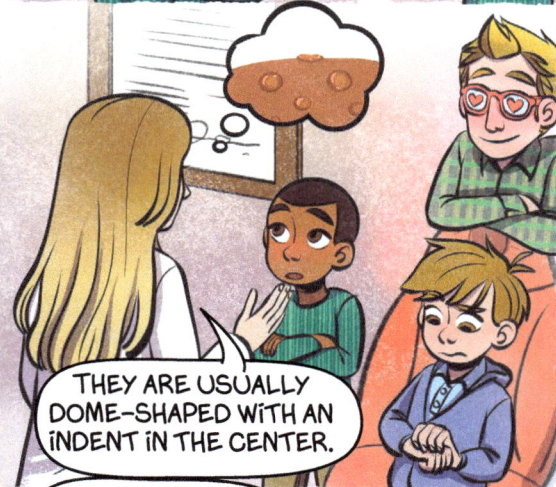

WHAT SHOULD I DO?

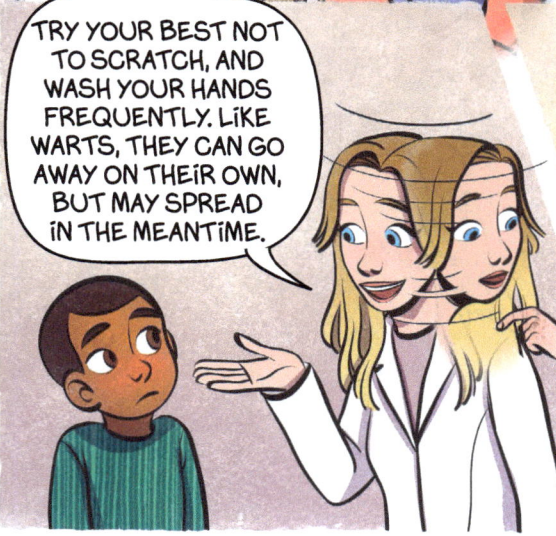

THEY ARE USUALLY DOME-SHAPED WITH AN INDENT IN THE CENTER.

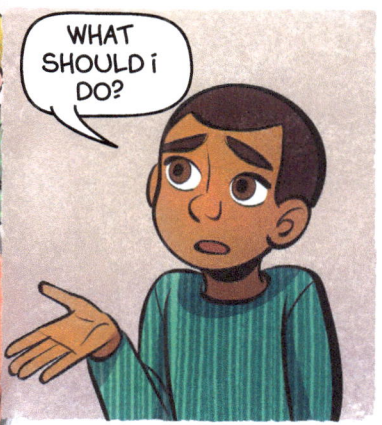

TRY YOUR BEST NOT TO SCRATCH, AND WASH YOUR HANDS FREQUENTLY. LIKE WARTS, THEY CAN GO AWAY ON THEIR OWN, BUT MAY SPREAD IN THE MEANTIME.

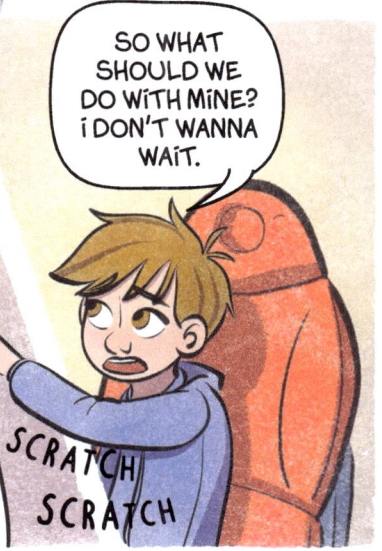

SO WHAT SHOULD WE DO WITH MINE? I DON'T WANNA WAIT.

SCRATCH

SCRATCH

THERE ARE **A FEW** WAYS TO TREAT WARTS AND MOLLUSCUM.

WE CAN **WAIT AND SEE** IF THEY GO AWAY ON THEIR OWN, BUT THAT CAN TAKE A LONG TIME.

SEEING THAT THEY'VE SPREAD AND BOTHERING YOU, I SUGGEST TREATING THEM.

WE CAN TRY **LIQUID NITROGEN**, WHICH IS A REALLY COLD SMOKY GAS THAT FREEZES THEM.

OR WE CAN PUT ON SOME **BLISTER BEETLE JUICE!**

Cantharidine

OR PINCH AND BURN THEM OFF. THESE CAN STING A BIT.

SPOOKY, SMOKY NITROGEN, BEETLES—SOUNDS COOL!

DID YOU KNOW THAT BLISTER BEETLE JUICE IS MADE BY AN ACTUAL BEETLE?

WOW, COOL! DOES IT HURT?

ONLY IF YOU LEAVE THE TREATMENT ON TOO LONG AND FORGET TO WASH IT OFF.

I would apply a drop of beetle juice painlessly onto each bump

And you'd leave it on for a few hours before washing it off at home.

It causes the skin to blister up and remove a piece or the entire wart.

I would see you again in a few weeks, it might take a few treatments to get rid of all of them.

WHAT IF I FORGET AND LEAVE IT ON TOO LONG?

SET AN ALARM!

GREAT IDEA! DAD CAN HELP REMIND YOU, TOO.

ON IT!

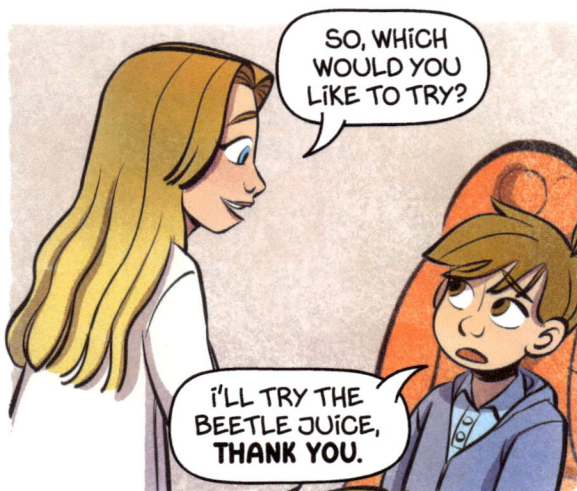

SO, WHICH WOULD YOU LIKE TO TRY?

OKAY, BUT BEFORE THAT, LET ME SHOW YOU THE LIQUID NITROGEN. IT'S PRETTY COOL.

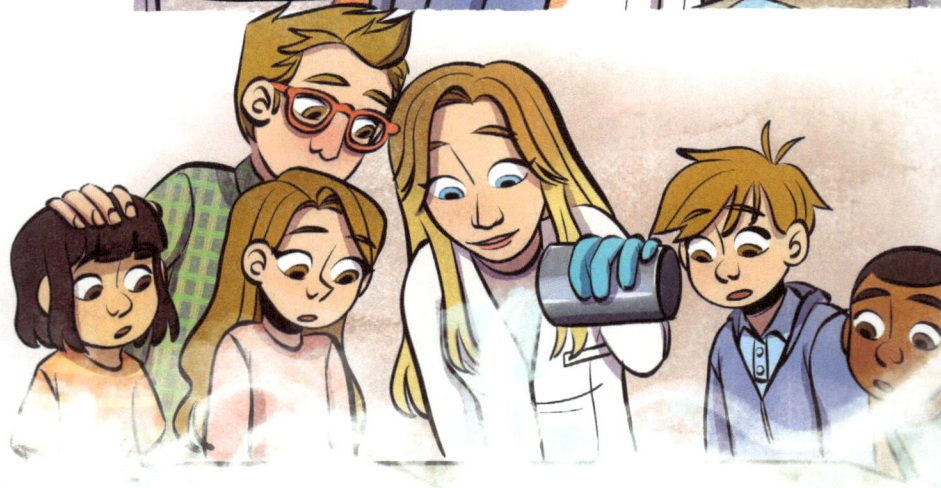

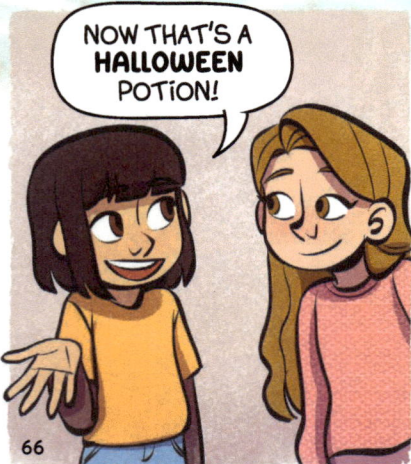

I'LL TRY THE BEETLE JUICE, **THANK YOU.**

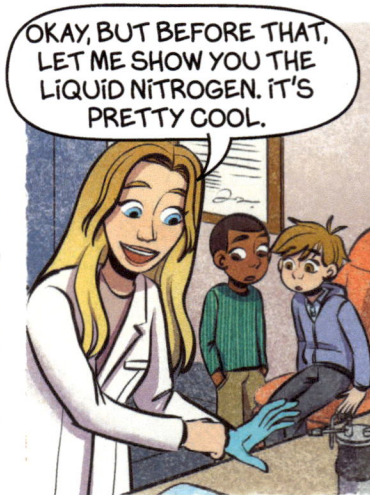

NOW THAT'S A **HALLOWEEN** POTION!

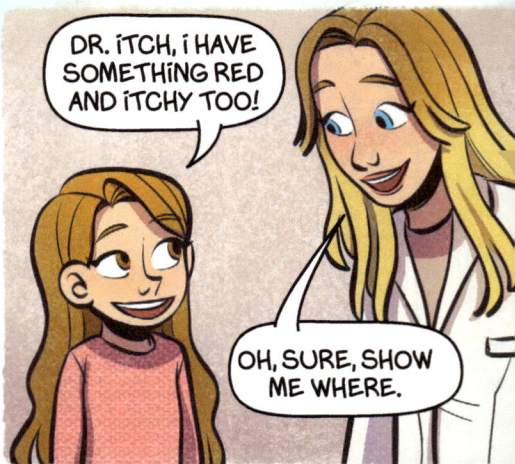

DR. ITCH, I HAVE SOMETHING RED AND ITCHY TOO!

OH, SURE, SHOW ME WHERE.

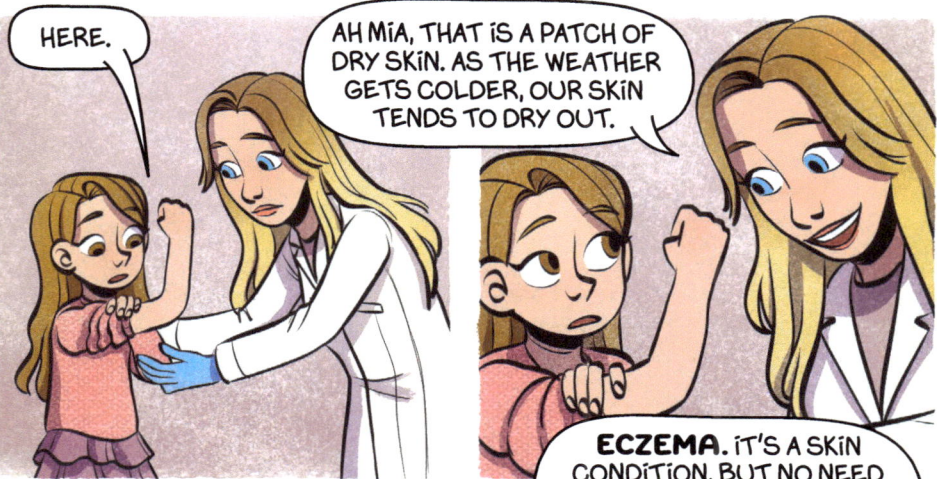

HERE.

AH MIA, THAT IS A PATCH OF DRY SKIN. AS THE WEATHER GETS COLDER, OUR SKIN TENDS TO DRY OUT.

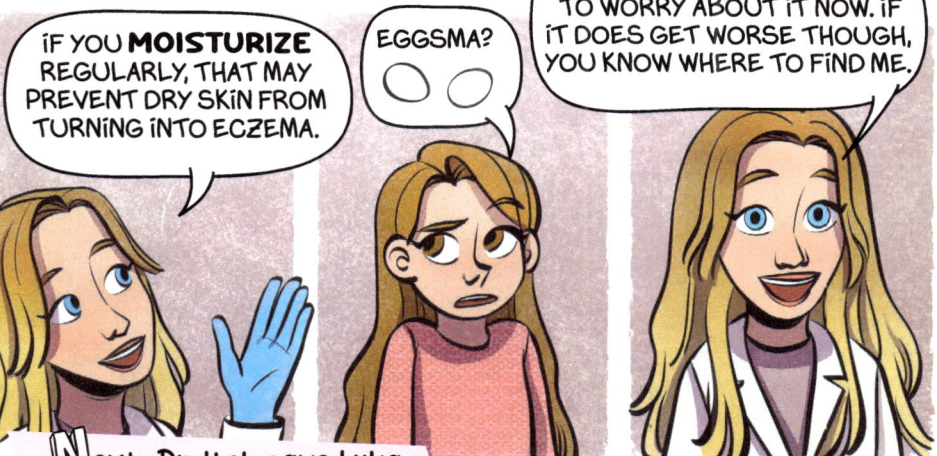

ECZEMA. IT'S A SKIN CONDITION, BUT NO NEED TO WORRY ABOUT IT NOW. IF IT DOES GET WORSE THOUGH, YOU KNOW WHERE TO FIND ME.

IF YOU **MOISTURIZE** REGULARLY, THAT MAY PREVENT DRY SKIN FROM TURNING INTO ECZEMA.

EGGSMA?

Next, Dr. Itch gave Luka his beetle juice treatment. He barely even complained.

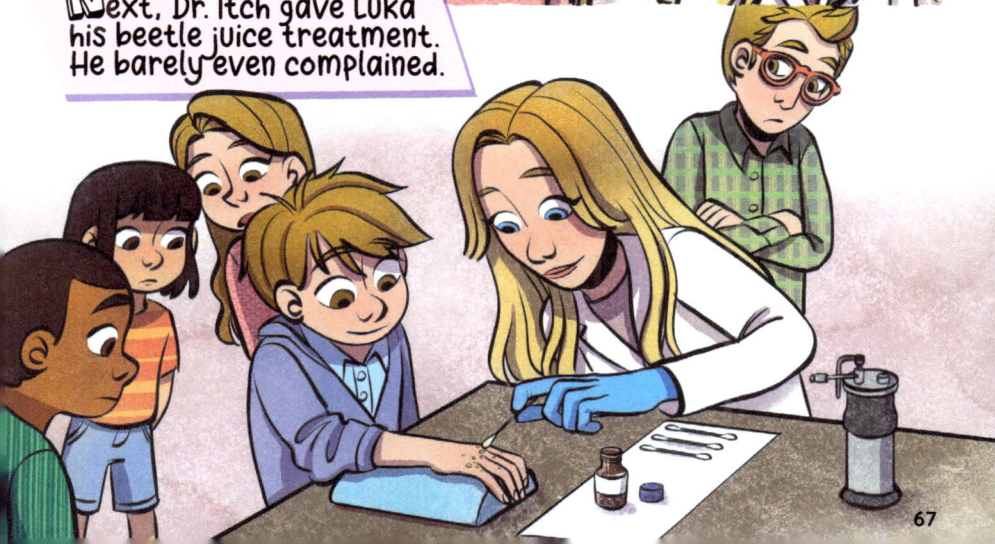

67

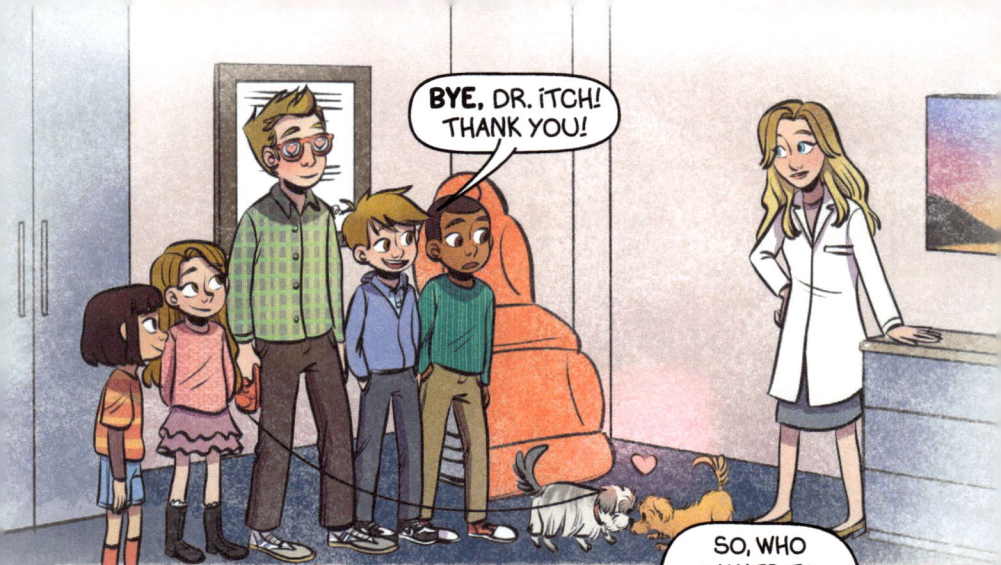

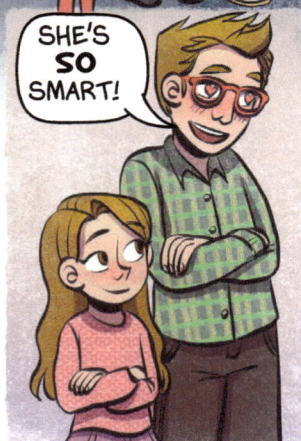

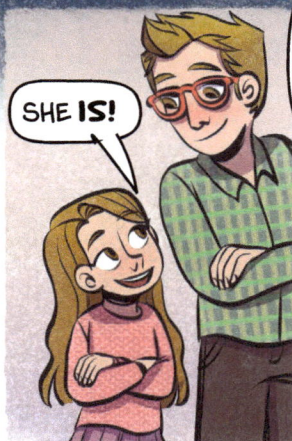

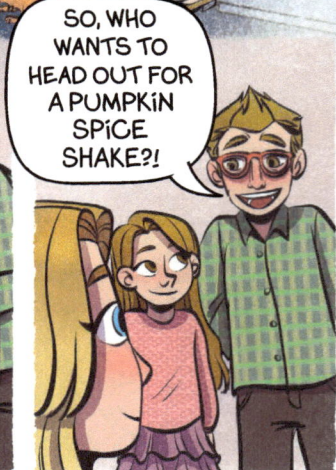

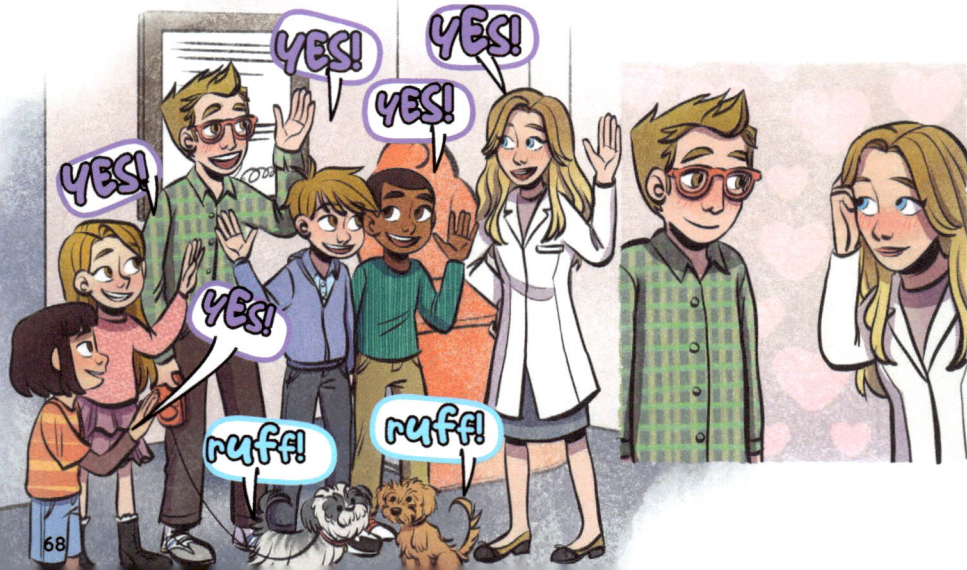

So, in the end, it was still a super spooky Halloween, between getting lost in the woods and making our first potion. I guess we're not witches after all, but Dr. Itch— I mean, Dr. Lazic— was there to save the day!

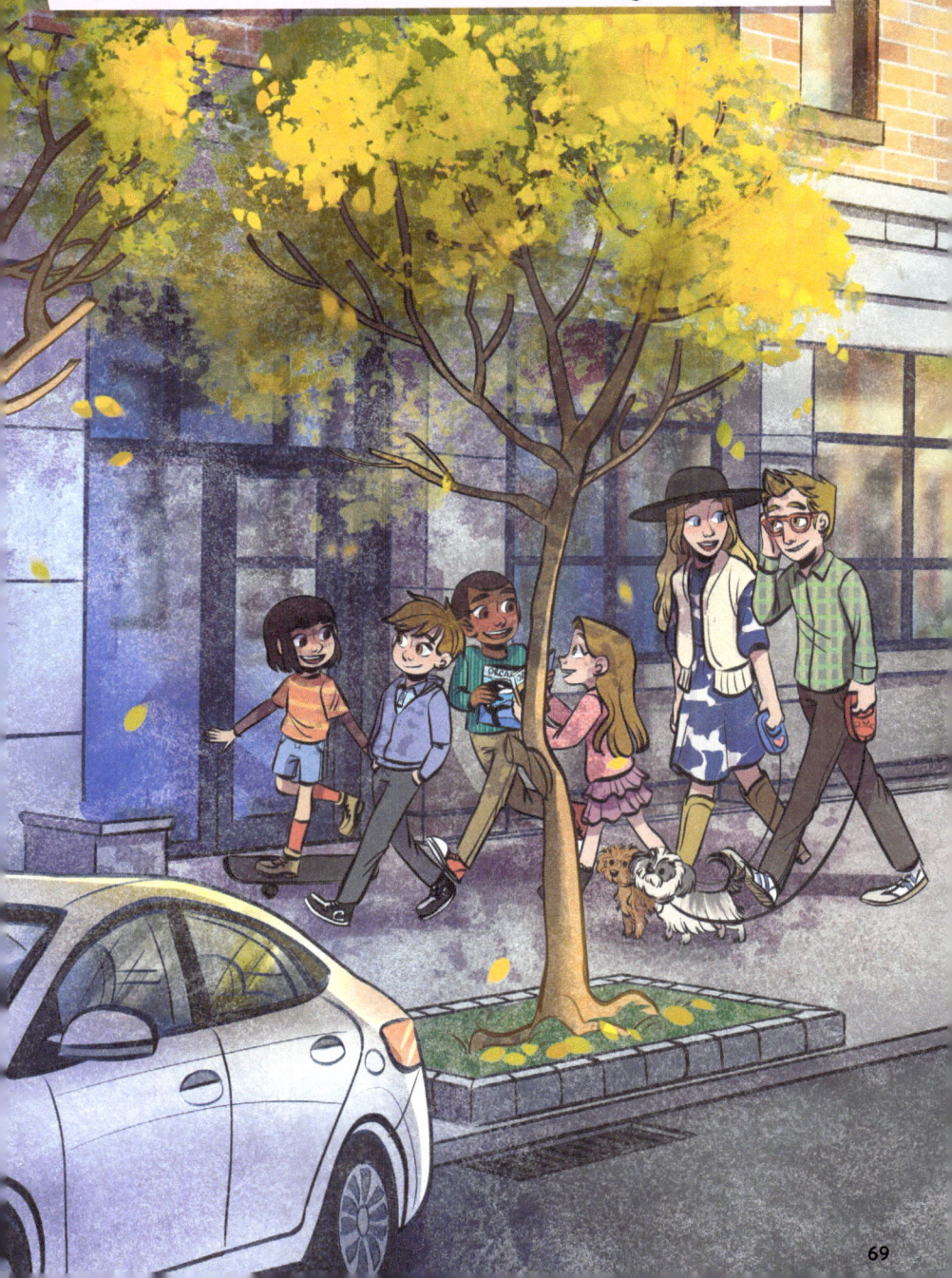

HOW TO TREAT AND PREVENT WARTS

Reference: www.aad.org

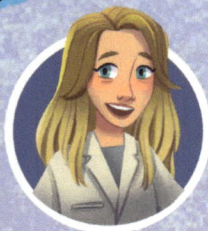

> IF SOMEONE IN YOUR FAMILY GETS A WART, YOU CAN HELP IT GO AWAY QUICKER AND PREVENT NEW WARTS FROM DEVELOPING!

SIX WAYS TO PREVENT WARTS

The virus that causes warts, human papillomavirus (HPV), spreads easily from person to person, and is found everywhere. By taking these dermatologist-recommended precautions, you can reduce the risk of getting warts:

1

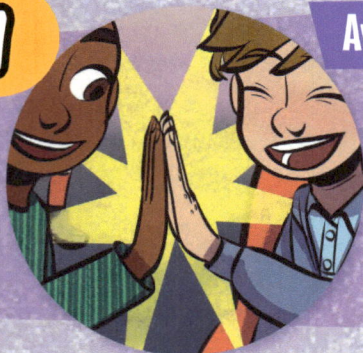

Avoid touching someone's wart.

HPV is contagious. It's possible for the virus to get inside your body through a cut or scratch (if you have one, keep it clean and covered!), which can cause a wart.

2 Don't share items that may be contaminated.

Make sure that everyone in your home has their own towels, razors, nail clippers, socks, and other personal items.

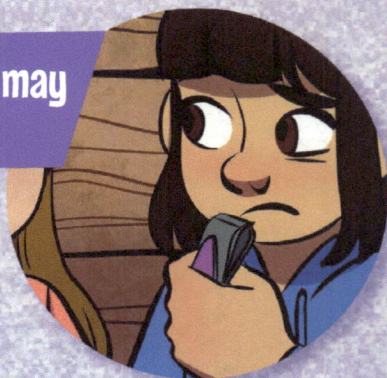

3 Wash your hands often.

Because HPV is so common, this helps to remove the virus from your skin.

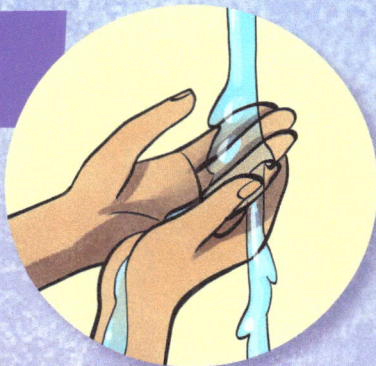

4 Prevent dry, cracked skin.

When skin is cracked and dry, it's easier for HPV to slip in through a crack in your skin, which could cause a wart. Moisturize if your skin is dry.

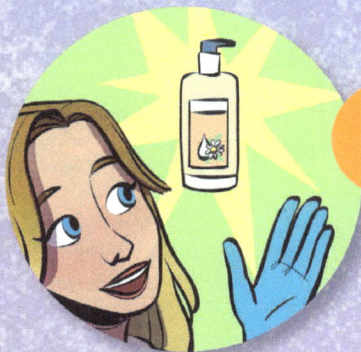

5 Stop nail biting and cuticle chewing.

When you bite your nails or cuticles, it causes sores and tears in the skin that are too tiny to see. These openings make it easier for HPV to get inside your body.

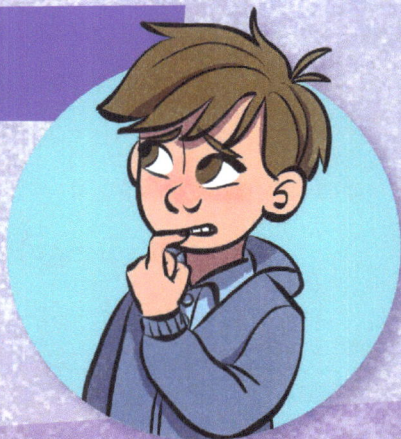

6 Wearing flip-flops can help prevent warts.

Wearing flip-flops or other shoes in moist areas, such as pool decks, public showers, and locker rooms can reduce your risk of developing warts on your feet.

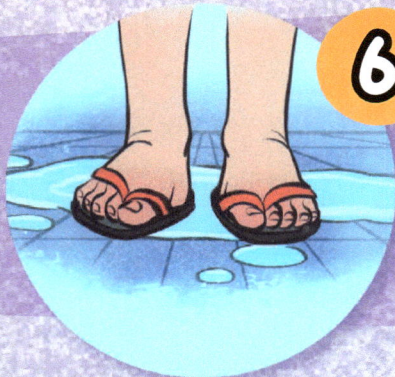

AT-HOME WART REMEDIES

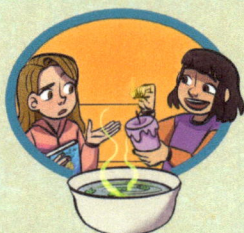

Your adults can help you try the following at home, before seeing a dermatologist:

1 Salicylic acid

This medicine is available without a prescription. It comes in different forms — a gel, liquid, or plaster (pad).

Apply salicylic acid to the wart every day.

Salicylic acid is rarely painful. If the wart or the skin around the wart starts to feel sore, you can take a break from the treatment for a short time.

It can take many weeks of treatment to see results, even when you do not stop treatment.

2 Other home remedies

Some home remedies are easy, such as covering warts with duct tape. Changing the tape every few days might peel away layers of the wart. Studies conflict, though, on whether duct tape really gets rid of warts.

Many people think certain folk remedies and hypnosis get rid of warts. Since warts may go away without treatment, it's hard to know whether a folk remedy worked or the warts just went away.

! ASK A DERMATOLOGIST IF YOU ARE UNSURE ABOUT THE BEST WAY TO TREAT A WART.

We hope that this book gives you an idea of how dermatologists treat warts (blister beetle juice, liquid nitrogen and all…). You now know what to expect if you need to see a doctor to treat your warts. If Luka could do it, so can you!

QUIZ

Courtesy of Ella Taft,
Class of 2027,
The Brearley School, NY

1. Where can warts be found on your body?

- **A** Hands
- **B** Feet
- **C** Elbows
- **D** All of the above

2. Which of the following is NOT a way to catch a wart?

- **A** Touch someone else's wart
- **B** Eat grapes or lemons
- **C** Walk barefoot at public pools
- **D** Touch your own wart

3. Which of the following is not a wart color?

- **A** Pink
- **B** Skin-colored
- **C** Brownish
- **D** Green

4. Which TWO of the following are NOT ways to treat a wart?

- **A** Scratch the wart
- **B** Blister beetle juice
- **C** Liquid nitrogen
- **D** Pick your nose

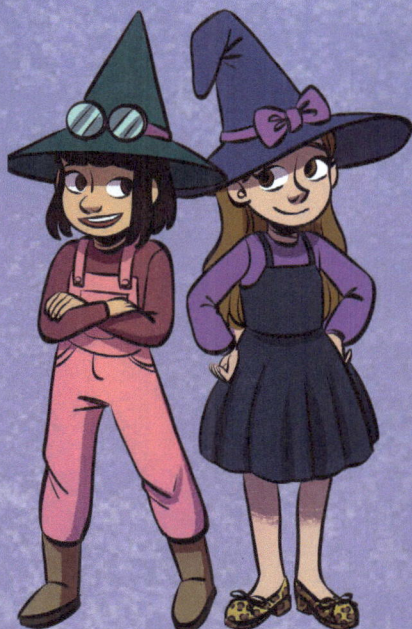

5. How long does blister beetle juice usually take to get rid of a wart?

- **A** Minutes
- **B** Days
- **C** Weeks to months
- **D** Years

Correct answers to all of the quiz questions are on the last page!

CROSSWORD PUZZLE

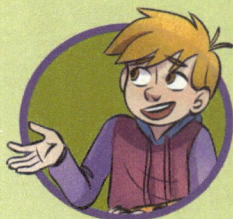

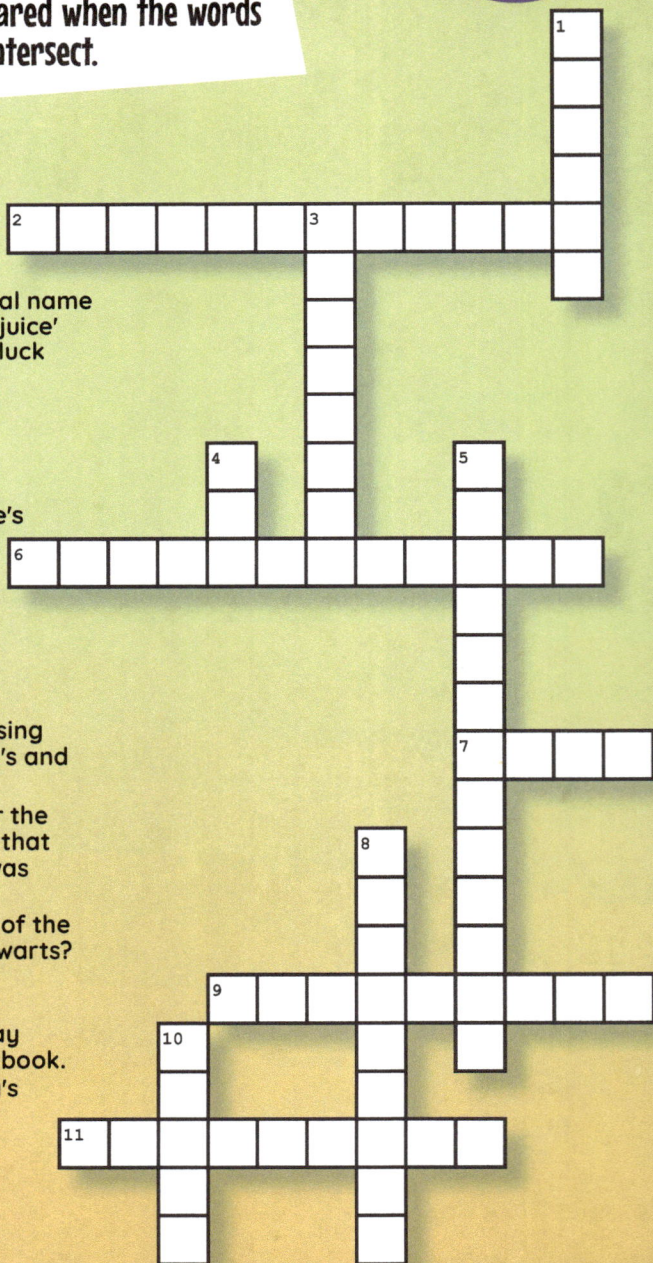

Use the clues to fill in the words above. Words can go across or down. Letters are shared when the words intersect.

ACROSS

2 What is the medical name for 'blister beetle juice' treatment? Good luck spelling this one!

6 The name of this book series.

7 A killer whale.

9 The name of Jude's skin condition.

11 The title of this book.

DOWN

1 What was the missing ingredient for Mia's and Anya's potion?

3 Do you remember the foreign language that the potion book was written in?

4 What is the name of the virus that causes warts?

5 A skin doctor.

8 The spooky holiday celebrated in this book.

10 The name of Luka's skin condition.

```
Z B R P Y U E T W K I T K B C
F H N D I K B B Y C R W G Z D
J P E N W I T C H E S C P E E
T O E I E V G Y V Z L M U R R
V T W U U E N C M X Z H S U M
B I O N Y F W Y O V Q C D T A
D O T N S I V O L T B E R N T
E N R R M T B M L H D E S E O
O J A C V J C P U L M N T V L
A V W V I R U S S Q A E R N O
X E A C T M C G C S W H A I G
K Q H S P C A K U E O N W K I
R R C K E L N Z M G F A V S S
L T I G S L D D R W P V F C T
P N K I H H Y B Y M R H B I X
```

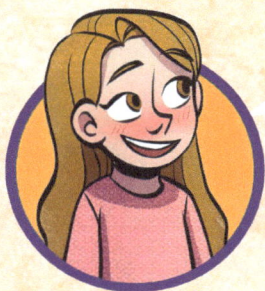

WORDSEARCH

Find the word in the puzzle. Words can go in any direction. Words can share letters as they cross over each other.

You can find more games and puzzles at

SKINVENTUREZ

skinventurez.com

SCAN ME!

@skinventurez

Witches
Potion
Virus
Molluscum
Warts
Halloween
Wartoween
Pumpkin
Candy
Dermatologist
Skinventurez

About this project

After practicing dermatology for over a decade in New York City, I was diagnosed with stage IV cancer and while on medical leave, I decided to finally write the children's books about skin I had always dreamed of writing.

I created a graphic novel series **SKINVENTUREZ** that promotes skin health via storytelling. While the first novel *The Sunscreaming Summer* emphasizes sun protection, this Halloween-inspired sequel Wart-o-ween educates kids about warts and other common viral growths and aims to reduce the stigma associated with them.

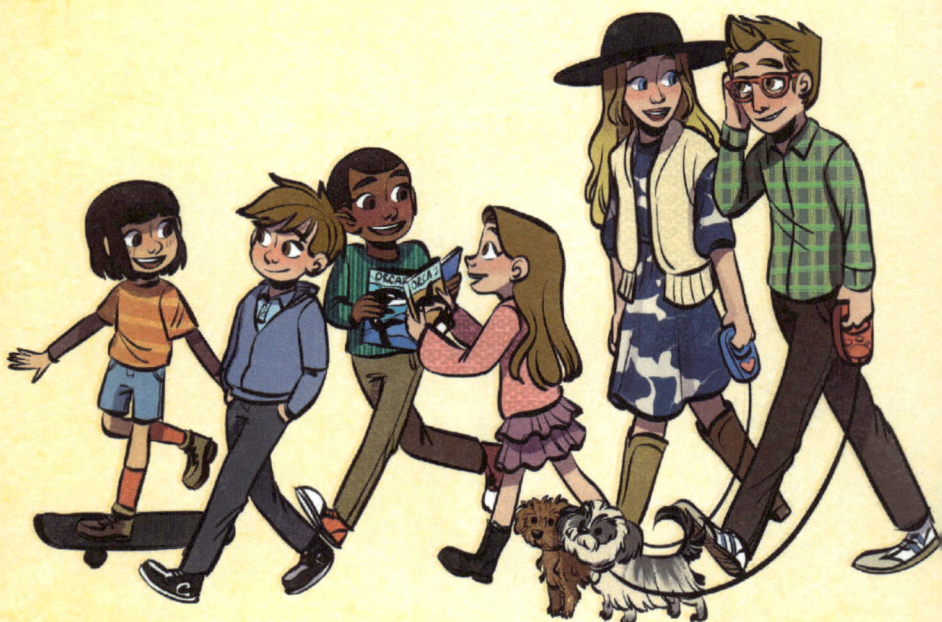

Here are the goals of this book:

- Normalize warts by teaching kids that warts are common and a part of growing up

- Encourage open communication by creating a safe space for kids to talk about their concerns and feelings about their warts

- Provide reassurance by letting kids know warts are typically harmless

- Offer treatment options and involve children in the decision-making process

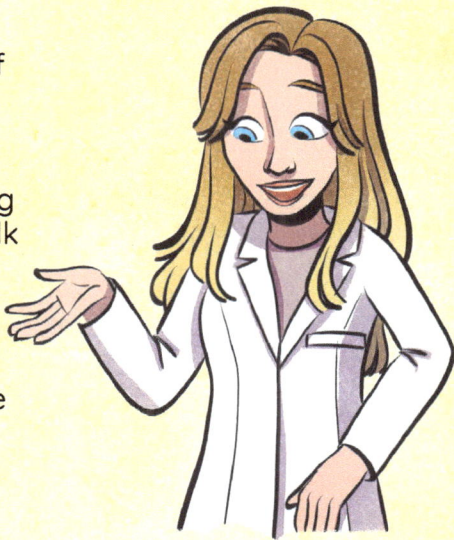

With future titles in the **SKINVENTUREZ** series highlighting conditions like eczema, acne and others, I hope to empower young readers to take control of their skin health and feel comfortable in their own skin.

Thank you for embarking on this journey with me!

About the Author

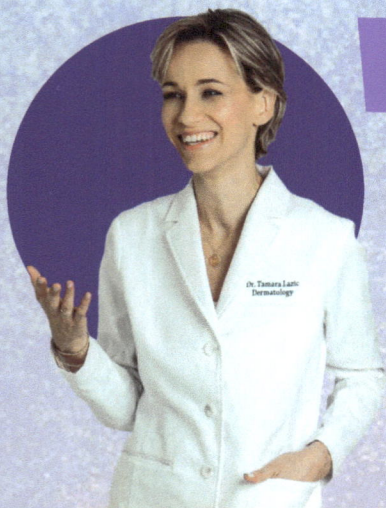

Dr. Tamara Lazic Strugar was born and raised in Serbia, and moved from her war-torn homeland to the US at the age of 18. She received her Bachelor of Science degree from UCLA where she graduated with highest honors and various awards, including the Tom Brokaw Award for Life Achievements. Dr. Lazic obtained two degrees from Yale University, completing both her medical school training and internship there. She went on to complete dermatology residency at Boston University's Roger Williams Medical Center, where she served as Chief Resident and received multiple awards for patient care and academic excellence. In 2012, she accepted an academic position at Mount Sinai's St. Luke's and Roosevelt Hospitals in New York City. She is an Associate Clinical Professor at Icahn School of Medicine at Mount Sinai and has published numerous dermatologic articles and book chapters.

@drlazicnyc
www.drtamaralazic.com

As a full-time dermatologist and mom of two young children, finding time to commit to the children's books she's always dreamed of writing was difficult. After being diagnosed with stage IV cancer in the spring of 2022, she took a break from clinical practice to undergo treatment and dedicated her spare time to writing the SKINVENTUREZ graphic novel series, using storytelling to teach kids about skin health.

When she isn't writing children's books or working on skincare consulting projects, and while still fighting cancer, Tamara enjoys spending time with her husband John and their children Mia and Luka, traveling the world every chance they get (including trips to Europe for cancer treatments). They split their time between New York City and Connecticut along with their dogs, Tito and Ginger. It's Tamara's hope that her young readers learn valuable lifelong health lessons from her book that stay with them long after the book is closed.

To learn more about Dr. Lazic, visit www.drtamaralazic.com or @drlazicnyc on Instagram.

About the Illustrator

Lea Embeli is a painter, illustrator and concept artist. She graduated from the Faculty of Applied Arts in Belgrade in the Department of Applied Painting, where she received her first Masters in Art degree. During her studies, she was awarded multiple scholarships such as the scholarship of the Ministry of Education, Science and Technological Development, as well as the Dositej scholarship from the Foundation for Young Talents.

She was also a recipient of various awards for academic excellence, and in 2021 she received a research scholarship

Photo by
Shintsubo Kenshu

:camera: **@leaem_illustration**

from the Japanese government to attend the University of Art in Tokyo, where she is currently working on her second Masters degree, this time in oil painting.

Apart from painting, in 2016 she began to illustrate books for various European publishers and worked in animation and concept art.

To learn more about Lea's work, visit her on Instagram @leaem_illustration.

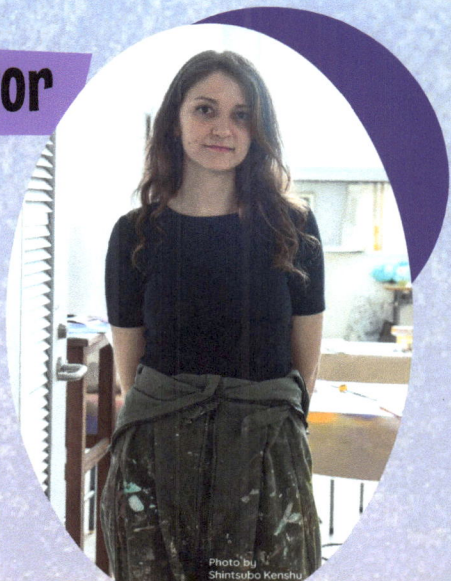

About the Designer

Biljana Mihajlović is an illustrator and graphic designer from Belgrade.

She graduated from the Academy of Applied Technical Studies in graphic design with a master's degree in book design.

She has been a member of the Association of Artists and Designers of Applied Art of Serbia (ULUPUDS), since 2021. She was the editor and illustrator of the magazine Let's Go Friends, and a proud author of children's illustrations published by domestic and

:camera: **@mihajlovic.biljana**

international publishers, such as IP Book, Magical Book , Creative Center, Odyssey, Little Bee, Freska and Klett.

She has numerous group and solo exhibitions and is the winner of several awards and recognitions in the field of illustration and graphic design.

Acknowledgements

MY FAMILY:

First and foremost, I would like to thank my family- my daughter Mia, son Luka and husband John ("Dad") for their love, support and inspiration. Mia, you are my #1 advisor and co-writer, this book series would not be what it is if it weren't for your endless imagination, creativity and attention to detail. Luka, your sense of humor (which I perhaps lack) was inspiring in creating the storyline and characters. John, you are the most supportive and loving husband and dad, thank you for not letting me give up on this journey, despite all the obstacles.

MY INTERNATIONAL TEAM:

Lea (Serbia/Japan)- I could not have asked for a more perfect illustrator, I knew it from the moment I saw your work online and hunted you down to join my project. Thank you for agreeing to embark on this journey with me, we have many more books to create together...two down, many more to go.

I would also like to thank my book designer Biljana (Serbia) who dived into our project in book #2, quickly found her way around and became an invaluable member of the team.

I am also thankful to our international publishers Kugli & Kugli (Croatia) and Makart (Serbia) for believing in the project and its mission.

And finally, I am thankful for every day on this Earth. To many more...

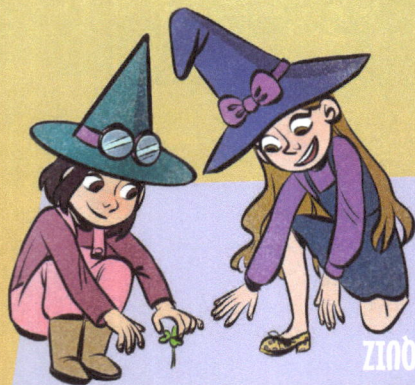

ANSWERS TO THE QUIZ

1 - D All of the above
2 - B Eat grapes or lemons
3 - D Green
4 - A & D Scratch the wart/pick your nose
5 - C Weeks to months

www.ingramcontent.com/pod-product-compliance
Lightning Source LLC
Chambersburg PA
CBHW041303290326
41931CB00032B/9